T0370394

Endorsements and Recommendations

"Simu Seaforth's 'Little Book of Qi' is a fascinating journey into both the ancient roots of Tai Chi and Qigong, as well as the awareness of the energetic nature of our bodies and the universe - a centering "inner awareness" more important in today's rapid change than at any time in human history." *William Douglas, Jr., author of "The Gospel of Science: Mind-Blowing New Science on Ancient Truths to Heal Our Stress, Lives, and Planet" (2nd EDITION, Jan. 1, 2022) and Founder of World Tai Chi and Qigong Day.*

"This book is the culmination of decades of experience and wisdom. From the esoteric to the practical key concepts from Qigong, Tai Chi and Daoism are interwoven through relatable stories, descriptions, and movement practices. A great read to all Qi cultivators." *Lori Furbush, former Chairperson, Board of Directors at National Qigong Association, teacher at Mindfulness-Based Stress Reduction (MBSR), Qigong, Yin Yoga, Reiki, and author of "Elemental Moves: Qigong Practices Inspired by Nature."*

"'Little Book of Qi,' is very engaging, weaving the history in with personal experiences and storytelling. It's absolutely perfect for beginners and has important depth for seasoned practitioners. It's a very important book to have!" *Shifu/Sensei Kore Grate, Executive Director/Head Instructor, Five Element Martial Arts and Healing Center, Minneapolis, MN. Executive Director at AWMAI, Association of Women Martial Artists Instructors.*

"I am happy to see Simu Janet Seaforth releasing this book to share her story and experience of how qi-cultivation has helped her life. Janet is an elder of the qi-cultivation community in Sonoma County, and I am eager to hear her perspective and wisdom garnered though decades of consistent practice." *Jacob Newell, Daoist priest, Nameless Stream, Old Oak School of Dao, author, and Stewardship Planner/Specialist Sonoma County Agricultural Preservation and for Open Space District.*

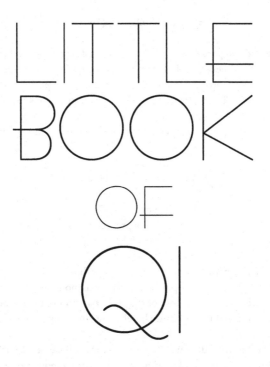

LITTLE BOOK OF QI

ENERGY FOR LIFE

JANET SEAFORTH

BALBOA.PRESS
A DIVISION OF HAY HOUSE

Balboa Press books may be ordered through booksellers or by contacting:

Balboa Press
A Division of Hay House
1663 Liberty Drive
Bloomington, IN 47403
www.balboapress.com
844-682-1282

Because of the dynamic nature of the Internet, any web addresses or links contained in this book may have changed since publication and may no longer be valid. The views expressed in this work are solely those of the author and do not necessarily reflect the views of the publisher, and the publisher hereby disclaims any responsibility for them.

The author of this book does not dispense medical advice or prescribe the use of any technique as a form of treatment for physical, emotional, or medical problems without the advice of a physician, either directly or indirectly. The intent of the author is only to offer information of a general nature to help you in your quest for emotional and spiritual well-being. In the event you use any of the information in this book for yourself, which is your constitutional right, the author and the publisher assume no responsibility for your actions.

Any people depicted in stock imagery provided by Getty Images are models, and such images are being used for illustrative purposes only. Certain stock imagery © Getty Images.

Print information available on the last page.

ISBN: 979-8-7652-2501-1 (sc)
ISBN: 979-8-7652-2504-2 (hc)
ISBN: 979-8-7652-2505-9 (e)

Library of Congress Control Number: 2022902976

Balboa Press rev. date: 06/03/2022

CONTENTS

ABOUT THE BOOK

The Little Book of Qi is written for anyone who wants to know more about the mysterious energy known as Qi and how it can be enhanced through Qigong and Tai Chi practice. The author connects insights developed by ancient Taoists, hermits, healers, and warriors over thousands of years. The book includes Buddhist teachings, feminism, and modern scientific understanding of ourselves and the universe. Janet shares memories of her own journey as a Tai Chi student growing in her practice. Her stories of working with her root teacher Sifu Nam Singh and other martial arts masters illuminate the special relationship students have with their teachers. Other stories take us into the exciting time at the nexus of the women's movement and the development of the martial arts on the west coast when women took their place as teachers and warriors.

Janet includes simple Qigong practices that allow the reader to experience the principles she teaches in each chapter. These practices are healing and restorative. They calm the mind and lighten the spirit.

ACKNOWLEDGEMENTS

This book was made possible by several dear friends and students. My deep thanks to Amy Neel, who suggested I write a book about Qi. Amy stuck with me through several drafts and offered essential edits for clarity. I am eternally grateful to Lynne Abels, a brilliant writing coach, who diligently and patiently helped me with every word on this epic journey. Lynne gave me the structural bones for this book, which combines personal stories, teachings of Chinese philosophy and history, and simple Qigong practices. She patiently inspired me to dig deep into my honest understanding and express it in words. I want to thank Susana Yavorsky, who read the draft and offered helpful suggestions and Jacqueline Gilman who helped prepare the manuscript. For the final magical touches, it was delightful to work with my wise and generous colleague, Marilyn Motherbear Scott, the bardic queen of the Mysteries.

I am ever grateful to Sifu Nam Singh, my beloved first teacher of Taoism, Qigong, Tai Chi, Chinese weapons, and herbal healing. I would also like to thank all teachers who have informed me over the past forty-five years. I spent several years training with Sifu Joe Deisher, and his teacher Master Chang I Chong. I especially treasure the women teachers and masters at Pacific Association of Women in the Martial Arts (PAWMA) including Wen Mei Yu, Pat Rice, Margaret Emerson, Kore Grate, and my Tai Chi sister, Sifu Michelle Dwyer. I also want to acknowledge the Aikido masters I have worked with, Sensei Michelle Benzamine Miki, Sensei Gayle Fillman, and Sensei Margie Leno. Thanks to Daniel Reid for his book, The Complete Book of Chi Gung.

In Sonoma County, I'm grateful to have studied with Sifu Joanne Stubblefield, her teacher Master Shu Dong Li, and many masters who participated in the United States Qigong Federation. It was at Master Li's Tai Chi Academy, I met teenager Sifu Justin Eggert. He is now a well-known World Martial Arts judge. I am forever grateful that Justin invited me to participate in the Wushu Championships in China in 2012.

I'm also grateful for Master Ming Tung Gu, who taught me his medical Qigong and Wisdom Healing Qigong. I also learned wonderful forms at the National Qigong Association, including Mathew Sweigart's Twelve Meridian form which you will find in this book.

I would like to express my gratitude to Louise Hay who gave me the mantra, "I trust and love the universe. Life itself supports me." It's why I choose Hay House and Balboa Press as my first publishers.

DEDICATION

To my students, who keep me inspired.
And my wonderful creative family.

INTRODUCTION

On the day of my graduation and induction into Dragon Tiger Mountain Temple, my teacher (or Sifu) gave me a statue from his altar. The white ceramic figure depicted one of the Eight Immortals revered by Taoists. My Sifu said the Immortal he gave me represents the historian and story teller. He was inspired to give it to me because I always carried a notebook and asked a lot of questions.

Forty years later I am fulfilling my mission to write down what I have found to be the most meaningful and beneficial teachings of Qigong, Tai Chi Chuan, and to explore the mysterious qualities of Qi itself.

I grew up in a working-class family in the north woods close to the Pacific Ocean. My mother was a devout Christian who believed, like Paul, that we should pray and meditate without ceasing. She was a dedicated Biblical scholar and believed in the healing power of the Holy Spirit. I was her "prayer partner" and witnessed many healings throughout my childhood. As I grew older, I became disillusioned with fundamentalist dogma and the guilt and fear it produced. I turned to the study of other religions, philosophy, and science to find the truth about how energy works.

At the time I started Tai Chi I was questioning many things in my life. The systems weren't working for me, my marriage had fallen apart, my spiritual life was shattered, and I was depressed and angry. Qigong and Tai Chi helped me find balance and clarity. My practice is a loyal companion and through years of training I have found my way to a meaningful, happy, healthy life.

I was fortunate to find a teacher who shared his understanding of the esoteric traditions of Tai Chi as well as the martial art aspect. Sifu Nam Singh studied with a student of Chen Man Ching with lineage from the Yang style. Sifu Nam Singh taught a family set he learned as a child in Taiwan. My Sifu is a medicine man. He is a Chinese herbalist, yogi and swordsman. He tells wonderful stories and keeps the traditions of a Taoist priest.

My purpose in writing this book is to share the best part of my life which is my relationship with this art form and to relate stories about how Qigong and Tai Chi evolved. I share my understanding of how the ancients began to question and discover the qualities of the life-force or vital energy, they called Qi. They diagramed it in symbols, categorized its elements and qualities, discovered its healing capacity, and created a choreography to dance with it. Qigong and Tai Chi are that dance. They have survived many centuries because they work. Qigong and Tai Chi are prescriptions that you give yourself through daily practice. It costs nothing but your time. The investment returns good health, long life, and happiness.

ONE

Before the Beginning

Qi is the energy that makes up everything in our universe. It is life force or vital energy in everybody and everything. Qi is a vibrating energy like electricity. It has an off and on quality, a yin/yang aspect. It is like the quanta in physics and chemistry, which is the minimum value of a physical property involved in an interaction.

**Qi is Everything.
Everything is made of Qi**

Character of Qi

The character for Qi in the original Chinese pictogram shows a vessel with the lid lifting. Qi is energy. The power of the boiling water makes things move.

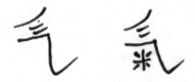

Chinese character for Qi by Janet Seaforth

The character implies ascending, vapor-forming clouds. In primitive times, it meant to offer a ritual prayer. In later times, the character shows a grain of rice cooking in the pot. It represents a kind of heat and force that makes things function and the nourishing quality of Qi.

Another translation of Qi is breath, or breath energy. Qi is made of yin and yang. Our inhale breath is yin, and the outgoing breath or exhale is yang.

Qi moves or runs in the body through invisible channels called meridians. Keeping these channels open and unblocked is a primary function of Qigong. For maximum Qi flow and to keep the channels open Qigong uses breath energy, postures, and stretches. Open flowing channels bring healing, harmony, and health to the body and mind.

Qigong is still practiced after thousands of years because it works!

In Traditional Chinese Medicine and acupuncture, there are twelve meridians associated with organs and there are also eight extraordinary meridians providing pathways of Qi. Qi is energy, gong is work or practice.

Qi is Energy.
Gong is Practice.

How my Practice Began

The year was 1975, a time of great experimentation with back-to-the-land skills and farming practices, old and new. One of the events that offered these activities was The Country Women's Festival. It was an all women's gathering deep in the woods of Mendocino County. The activities included: sheep shearing and tanning, gardening, and cooking, tuning up our cars and changing our own oil. We learned to use power tools, how to run our own business, and the art of self-defense.

My sister Caron, our daughters Bridget and Shiloh, and my partner Sue went to the festival to learn skills and connect to other independent women. Like many women there, Caron and I were single moms. We brought our girls, ages five and seven, with us.

As we were entering the camp with our backpacks on our back, we noticed women scurrying and laying out blankets in a small meadow not far from the main lodge. Sue asked a woman nearby, "What's going on?" The woman told her "A woman is giving birth." There were midwives at the festival who were helping her. Two women fiddle players were playing slow, calming, and haunting melodies which

3

became faster as the birth progressed. The musicians were attuned to the mother's energy. A crowd of women stood around the edges completely surrounding the mother and the midwives. By the time the baby was born, we were all crying with joy and amazement.

After a communal dinner at the lodge, we got settled in our cabins. I was concerned about how our girls felt about witnessing the birth of a human baby. They were used to seeing our goats give birth, but I wanted to know if they had any questions or if they felt disturbed by the event. They assured me they were ok and that they liked the fiddle music.

In the morning a martial arts training was held in the meadow. The instructor was Betty Braver, a brown belt in Shotokan Karate. She taught us the basics of how to defend ourselves from attack. Betty was a nurse and had seen many women suffer from rape and domestic abuse. Perhaps this is why she was determined to teach women to fight back. Betty asked all the women at the festival to make a commitment to ourselves and each other to learn the art of self-defense.

She had us raise our fist above our heads and promise we would learn to protect ourselves from any abuse. We took the pledge, "I will protect myself, and I refuse to be a victim!" We practiced simple strikes and blocks. Working in pairs, one woman would punch at her partner and the other woman would catch the strike, blocking it with her arm. I woke up the next morning with big bruises on my forearms. I wanted to learn to defend myself, but I didn't want to get hurt.

After breakfast in the old Mendocino Woodlands lodge, I stepped out onto the stone porch and noticed two women in the distance on a small meadow at the edge of the giant redwoods doing something together that I'd never seen before. They were moving very slowly, each appeared to have an invisible ball between her hands that she would turn and move in different directions. They moved in perfect unison. It was enchanting, and for me it was love at first sight. I wanted to do that! I went up to the women after they had completed their strange dance and asked them what they were doing. "Tai Chi," they said. They told me this beautiful art in motion was also a martial art.

I promised myself to find a Tai Chi teacher when I got back home. Advocates of the hard arts like Karate or Kung Fu didn't think Tai chi was a serious martial art, but I was determined that Tai Chi would fulfill the self-defense promise I made to Betty.

The full name of the beautiful dance I witnessed at the Country Women's Festival is Tai Chi Chuan. Tai Chi means Supreme Ultimate and Chuan means fist. It is known as the fist of self-containment. Chuan signifies refusing to be a victim and to taking responsibility for our life. This powerful martial arts practice sets a deep intention to respect ourselves and be responsible for our choices. We recommit to this Chuan every time we bow in at the beginning of our class and at the beginning of the form when we make that fist of self-containment.

**Chuan the fist of self-containment
implies the oath, "I take responsibility for
myself, and I refuse to be a victim."**

Tai Chi Chuan is about eight hundred years old. Qigong is said to be five thousand years old. Qigong originates from a time before writing. How did it survive all these centuries? With thousands of years of continuous history, China is one of the oldest civilizations in the world. Its culture honors its ancestors through rites and practices which keep alive the legends of its beginning. Stories and practices have been passed down through generations of shamen healers, energy workers, Traditional Chinese Medicine (TCM) practitioners and historians. Many versions, methods and forms of Qigong are practiced today. These practices have survived not only because of tradition but because of their profound and documented health benefits.

The Way of the Wu

**China is one of the oldest living
cultures in the world.
It embodies almost four thousand
years of dynastic rule.
Before the dynasties, there was the Wu.**

Chinese archeologists and historians write about the people of Wu who lived in the time of matriarchy about 5,000 to 10,000 years ago. Nomadic hunter gatherers started planting crops and domesticating animals about 10,000 years ago. The Wu lived in the lower reaches of the Yellow River where the soil was fertile. They were farming people organized around agriculture. It is said the people of the Wu did a ceremonial dance called Da Wu. The great dance was done to heal, restore balance in nature, and strengthen the people.

The women shamen and tribal leaders would communicate with the powers of heaven, earth, and humanity. They led "dances" to ward off disease, regulate breathing, and balance energy. The shamen also performed ritual dances to bring rain in times of drought and stop flooding. They began to develop herbal knowledge to preserve good health. This is the beginning of Qigong and Traditional Chinese Medicine.

This early spiritual practice of connecting to the spirit world influenced the later dynastic rule and its determination by the "Mandate of Heaven." Many references say the practice started in the Zhou Dynasty; however, other research suggests it was from Neolithic times. In the Zhou Dynasty, The Mandate of Heaven meant an emperor was sufficiently virtuous to rule. If he didn't fulfill his obligations, then he lost the Mandate and the right to be emperor.

The first legendary "kings" of China were from the Hsia or Xia period. They were called "Sons of Heaven." They were thought to be direct descendants from the Sky God or Thunder God, who was their heavenly parent. The most famous was Yu the Great who managed to divert water and decrease the flooding in the Yellow River. He was seen as a true Son of Heaven and born of a virgin.

The first historic ruler of China in the Bronze Age was T'ang. According to legend, he was born of a mother made pregnant by a bird's egg that fell from heaven. Even the men of Zhou had their own revered mother, distinct from the deified mother of the Shang. The story goes, his mother had stepped into the foot-print of a huge, divine being and bore the totemic ancestor of the Zhou line of kings. (*From the series Great Ages of Man, on China.*)

The Wu lived in a time of oral tradition. The oldest written record of the Wu is from the Shang Dynasty, 1600 BC to 1046 BC. Wu is found scratched into bones and shells that come from that time. "Wu" represented a living person, tribe, place, territory, or a shaman. Men shamen were called Xi, and women Wu.

In prehistoric times, women were honored for their birth-giving power. The first art depicts fertility Goddesses. The earth was honored because it gave us sustenance. The sky was honored as giving light and consciousness. When the written word came into use, so did the patriarchy. Women's place of power slowly diminished. Women were discouraged from being shamen and the word Wu came to imply witchcraft, with negative connotations even though the practice of divination was central to society throughout the dynastic rule. By the time of the Zhou, women were secluded at home and men conducted business outside the home. "Women weave, and men plow" was the motto of the Zhou.

Nu Wa and Fuxi

The Wu taught through stories. Indeed, the Chinese are still very fond of telling and listening to stories by professional story tellers. One creation story tells of Pangu who created the earth and the sacred mountains with his body after being born from the great cosmic egg. They also tell of the Goddess Nu Wa, (NuKua or Nu Gwa) who created people in a way similar to our Judeo-Christian story. Nu Wa was lonely, so she made men and women from yellow clay. It is said she created the first people by hand, but then to be more efficient she used a paint brush. As she breathed on the clay figures, they came to life.

It is said, the people multiplied and lived happily on the earth until great storms and fires threatened their existence. Nu Wa came to the rescue and repaired the hollows in heaven that had sent the heavy rains, and she killed the Black Dragon that had brought the storms. Then she stabilized the earth with a tortoise that she had captured.

The tortoise is famous for being the foundation of creation in many cultures. The Native Americans of Pohaten territory (Virginia) also believed creation began on the back of a turtle when Nokomis swung down from heaven on grape vines (possibly a symbol for the Tree of Life). With the help of swan wings, she came to Turtle Island, the name Native Americans use for their land. In this western version the turtle gives his back as a foundation for soil that beaver, muskrat and others bring to make land for humanity. The solid ground made it possible for the great Nokomis to descend bringing with her the Tree of Life. One wonders how these myths may have traveled, considering the common threads they share.

Nu Wa is depicted in paintings and sculptures from the great art of the Tang Dynasty with her consort the first king of the Chinese people, Fuxi. This may signify the time when the institution of marriage was created. The two are depicted with their lower bodies as two snakes intertwined like a caduceus. In their hands they hold a compass and a carpenter's square. They are considered the architects of the Chinese people, their culture, and the ancestors of humankind.

Fuxi lived in Henan province about 4,000 years ago and proclaimed himself as the first monarch. His Kingdom extended to the east coast in the first dynasty called the Xia (Hsia). Fuxi is credited with creating the symbol of the Eight Directions or Ba Gua. Legend says Fuxi was inspired by contemplating the patterns on the back of a tortoise.

In the thirteenth century Chang San Feng created Tai Chi based on the Ba Gua. By this time the Ba Gua had developed into the I Ching and a whole Confucian relationship of family positions.

Three Reasons to Learn Tai Chi

Tai Chi is mainly practiced for good health. The second reason is for meditation. The third reason is for self-defense. These three apparent differences are often integrated. For example, Tai Chi and Qigong are used as self-defense against stress and disease through moving meditation. Practitioners of Tai Chi and Qigong believe we are protected from disease by helping to cleanse the body of impurities by gentle movement.

In Tai Chi the whole body moves in alignment and the movements are synchronized with the breath. This brings harmony to all the body systems. Tai Chi is often called medicine in motion. Tai Chi and Qigong help the body process the medicine and food that we ingest. They calm the nerves and inspire a peaceful exhilaration.

I am forever grateful to have found Qigong and Tai Chi Chuan. This ancient practice not only filled my need for a martial-arts practice, it gave me emotional healing through meditation and physical relief from a pre-arthritic condition. At twenty-nine years old I was suffering from swelling, stiffness, and pain in my hands and lower back. I had been a potter working for hours throwing clay and creating sculpted goblets and vases as my way of making a living. I was in severe pain and anxious that I would have to give up the work I loved. Tai Chi allowed me to continue in my chosen career for many years.

The most important reason to do Tai Chi is for good health. Its gentle movements massage every joint and organ in the body. It calms the nerves and reduces stress. It helps the heart to push the blood to every cell of the body. The practice of Tai Chi has great power to refresh and rejuvenate our body.

Because of the slow movement, concentration and coordination with the breath, Tai Chi becomes a meditation. Qi is often called "life-breath energy". Our life is framed by the first and last breaths we take. Our breath is a powerful resource. Breathing deeply helps us relax, which helps the body to heal.

Our life is framed by the first and last breath we take.

Qigong has many meditation stances and various standing, sitting, and moving forms. Tai Chi Chuan is an elegant form of Qigong. These forms bring the mind into service of the body. With every movement the body, mind and spirit are brought into harmony. Daily practice strengthens our body, clears and calms our mind, and comforts and awakens our spirit. It is truly an alchemy that changes discord into harmony.

The martial aspect is the least important reason to learn Tai Chi. But it is important to the form because it defines the shape of the postures. Knowing the martial applications refines the form. The viability of the movements is tested by the martial arts postures. If your arm is too straight or too bent, you will not be as effective in a push. The Qi won't flow. You can test the shape of your form by pushing against a partner.

PAWMA

(Pacific Association of Women in Martial Arts)
Women in the Martial Arts

It was not easy to be a woman martial artist in the 1970's. The schools were male dominated. Most dojos didn't want to train women, because they thought the women would get hurt and disrupt the male camaraderie. The few women practitioners were wives or daughters of male martial artists.

Betty Braver organized the first "Women in the Martial Arts Camp" in the Sierra foothills in 1977. She invited women martial arts teachers and their students from the Bay Area, Sacramento, Southern California and from the area around Eugene, Oregon. One hundred women of various martial arts styles gathered for four days in the sweet smell of the sugar pines over the Labor Day weekend.

Betty Braver greeted the Tai Chi contingent at the first PAWMA camp by holding up her hand, palm out, and making circular motions in the air saying, "I know Tai Chi. It's circles, circles, circles!"

Most of the women looked tough. They didn't wear make-up, some were loud, some mysteriously silent. They came in with big, oddly shaped bags containing swords and staves and other weapons. At orientation the women were cautious, untrusting of other styles. Some seemed very arrogant. I wasn't sure what I had gotten myself into.

I was relieved that my Tai Chi sister Michelle Dwyer had come with me. We call each other sisters because we trained together for many years. I'd met Michelle the previous year when I joined Sifu Nam Singh's Tai Chi classes. We were both committed to learning, so we went. Michelle had sewn black cotton Tai Chi outfits for us trimmed with a royal blue border. We also took the swords we'd purchased to practice a graceful form we were learning from our Sifu, Nam Singh.

At PAWMA all the women were assigned to groups within their own style. Michelle and I were assigned to work with a Tai Chi teacher from L.A. There were about fifty Karate women and three in the Tai Chi category. No one knew what to do with us. We were an anomaly, because Tai Chi was so slow and soft and didn't look very martial. We didn't know how to fit in, but the training sharpened our skills and tested our mettle.

We took three workshop–classes a day and at night one-hundred women would eat dinner together. After doing the dishes and cleaning up and pushing the dining tables and benches to the walls, there would be a free-form workout in the great hall. Two or three rings would form of women sparring together with the fireplace roaring at the end of the lodge.

It was fascinating to see so many different forms and schools. Each school had its own uniform. The karate schools were attired in crisp white gis with their kimono style lapel and their belts tied in the fashion of their school. The judo women were usually larger women with looser gis. The Aikido teachers were mysterious, bare foot, wearing white gis with long black wide legged pants called hakamas. Some of the Kung Fu women stood out wearing bright silks with gold fringe which flashed when they demonstrated their katas at the Saturday night performance. They'd run, jump, and cartwheel as they broke stacks of pine boards. I was gleefully impressed. The gung fu school from Eugene led by a woman named Rita was thrilling to witness. They grappled and showed their stamina with routines that comprised kicking, punching and then dropping to the ground and moving across the hardwood floors of the great hall on their bellies. They looked like combat soldiers crawling towards an enemy. They wore black gis that were tattered from abuse.

The suspicion at the beginning of camp soon turned to curiosity and fascination as the women trained and sparred with each other. The orderly karate punch matched with the judo throw. Different schools and styles paired off to explore and test their best techniques. By the end of the long weekend, we learned to be more effective in our movements and our ability to concentrate improved.

There was a lot of laughter and hollering amid an occasional "kiai." The kiai is a loud guttural shout that we all practiced in several of the classes. It was strange at first but soon we could identify who was fighting from the definitive sound. Kiai echoed through the air from the rings of sparring both inside the lodge and out on the dirt under the pines or in the playing field. It was a war cry that came from the belly when a throw or a blow was administered. The women put their all into it.

I'll never forget the excitement of those first camps. Pacific Association of Women in the Martial Arts grew out of the success of those first few years. PAWMA has been a great training ground for many women with annual camps from Seattle to Los Angeles. The Tai Chi contingent grew to match the other martial arts in number. Teachers and masters from China were brought to teach at the camps, which benefitted all of us. The twenty camps that I attended have influenced me as much as any other teacher throughout my forty years of training. I am forever grateful to Betty Braver and Women in the Martial Arts.

Modern Qigong and Tai Chi Chuan

The communists took control of China in 1949. All the arts were transformed into the service of building a new China. Many Tai Chi masters left the country. The term "Qigong" was used to describe ancient physical energy practices, without any religious connotations. In 1956, China began to bring Qi Gong, Tai Chi and Gung Fu back into public practice. In the 1980's charismatic qigong healers and masters emerged, including Falun gong. Falun gong became the largest Qigong organization in China, rivaling the 70 million people of the Chinese Communist Party. It became resistant to the state and was banned.

The martial arts are again presented as health or gymnastic exercises and purposely devoid of any spiritual content. These arts are now called Wu Shu, which means "martial art."

In 1977 my Tai Chi teacher Sifu Nam Singh took several members of our Tai Chi class to the first performance in the United States of the Wushu team from China. The great performance was held at the Cow Palace in San Francisco. Thousands of people attended, most of them local Chinese, to watch the amazing show. The Chinese team demonstrated tremendous skills, especially in the use of weapons. There were many kinds of staff and sword routines and even flying stars. There was an older man who broke a block of granite that looked like a tomb stone with his head. Women twirling swords leapt so high into the air they looked like they were flying. Jet Li, the famous movie actor, was just a boy at the time and part of the Wushu team. We were all awestruck. One man lying flat on his back whipped a long chain under his entire body while lifting himself off the floor, as if by levitation. The performance seemed to be beyond the limit of human possibilities.

There are many Tai Chi forms, but the most popular Tai Chi form in the world today was created in 1956. It was called the Peking 24 Form and was designed by four masters and promoted by the government. It is now called the Beijing 24 Form or simply Tai Chi 24 Form. It is the standard competition form, and it takes about five minutes to perform. The Tai Chi 24 form is the most popular short form in the world.

Tai Chi is recognized by its slow, even, continuous movements. It is often practiced outside, in nature, either individually or by groups of practitioners. In the thirteenth century, the founder of Tai Chi, Chang San Feng, designed thirteen basic postures, which flow one into the next seamlessly. The original movements he created have evolved into the many lovely forms that exist today.

Lineage is important in the martial arts. When Tai Chi practitioners meet, one of the first questions asked is, "Who is your teacher?" My first Tai Chi teacher, Sifu (teacher) Nam Singh, learned the Dragon Tiger Mountain form at a boy's school in Taiwan. It was created by the grandmaster Cheng Man-ching as a special "family set" designed for that school. I don't know the name of the school, only that my teacher was taught by a student of the famous Cheng Man-ching.

Cheng Man-ching left China after the Cultural Revolution that forbade Qigong or Tai Chi practice. He moved to Taiwan and eventually came to New York in 1964. He is famous for popularizing Tai Chi in the United States. Cheng Man-ching died March 26, 1975. Out of respect for the Grand Master, Sifu brought black arm bands to class for us to wear on that day.

Wuji

Wuji is a fundamental practice of standing in stillness and alignment. Ideally every Tai Chi form begins with Wuji. The word Wuji is translated as not doing or doing nothing. The classic statement, *"Out of Wuji comes Tai Chi, out of nothing comes something,"* refers to the generative power of Wuji. When we are relaxed and still, we feel the subtle yang electromagnetic energy that surrounds us, and we allow the harmonizing Qi to flow through us. Wuji is a return to stillness that is essential to the act of creation. Sifu would say, "Let yourself be empty. Emptiness is like turning on the TV but without getting a picture. It's on, the juice is flowing, but there's no content." He also said, "The stance of Wuji is like being a big bell that is silent but has the potential for ringing."

Out of Wuji Comes Tai Chi

Wuji is a yin state. Yin is still, dark, and empty. From this clean slate or empty container, the yang energy of movement and light can emerge.

Wuji can be frightening to a person who is used to constant activity. If we can overcome our resistance and stay centered, our fears pass, and we are stronger for it. We begin to trust the process of letting thoughts come up and gently letting them go, like clouds streaming across a big blue sky. Our anxieties that make us want to run or fight often find resolution without action. Standing still, being in the moment, seeking no change in our outward physical state, we become witness to the invisible changes in our mind and allow the necessary internal action of our physical body to return to homeostasis.

Restoration to wholeness is a natural process when we relax in the stillness of Wuji. Wuji makes way for this transformation. In the dark, still, quiet place of dreaming, great ideas can spring forth from the subconscious mind. Some of the greatest creativity comes when a person is just waking from sleep. Einstein famously said, "Imagination is more important than knowledge." Many of his ideas and understanding came from intuition, inspiration, and feelings he experienced before he set them into equations and words. Once he dreamt of a sled going down a snowy slope so fast that everything around him changed. This dream led to the principle of relativity and the qualities of the speed of light. Niels Bohr won a Noble Prize for his work on the structure of the atom which he saw in a dream. The creative spark of imagination can seed a thought into a theory or invention from a dark, still, space.

In our practice we begin with Wuji to rid ourselves of outside noise and inner turmoil. We open to the soft state of aligned relaxation where we can be sensitive to the subtle qualities of movement. In this state of still presence our body is at a heightened ability to heal and to understand. When we practice Wuji before our Tai Chi form, we develop the trust that makes our Tai Chi more powerful.

With relaxed awareness we can be more effective in our movement and understanding.

The heightened awareness in the state of Wuji is similar to the understanding in the Ayurvedic science of ancient India. Dr. Deepak Chopra relates in his book <u>Quantum Healing</u> that Ayurveda means science of life. It is based on a belief that the body is created out of consciousness. The body and mind are intricately one system. It is understood in Ayurveda that "all that exists around me is part of myself." In qigong we feel this as a Qi field. We are in a sea of Qi.

In Ayurvedic medicine, Chopra says the material body is a river of atoms, the mind is a river of thought. What holds them together is a river of intelligence. This intelligence is a rich field of our inner space that exerts a powerful influence on us. Intelligence is found in every cell of our body. Each cell correlates its messages with trillions of other cells. It participates in thousands of chemical exchanges every second. The DNA carried in the cells are the record of life and of our ancestors. If we want to navigate the field of intelligence, we must learn about it in the very depths of our being, "where the silent witness inside us waits."

The primal energy of creation is called pure harmonious Qi or Yuan Qi. A quality of Yuan Qi is Loving Light. This can be seen as a universal intelligence or consciousness. When we are in stillness, we can connect to our own consciousness, to the universal consciousness and the energy of love. This energy is peaceful, forgiving, and

21

healing. When we stand in Wuji we can feel the state of grace and the purity of the oneness that connects all. We enter into a vast openness when we realize we are part of the whole universe. The great void before the beginning of time and space was the womb of all creation. We think of it as formless, undifferentiated energy, that holds all the possibilities of creation.

We are part of unfolding evolution from the time of the Big Bang 13.7 billion years ago. The elements that are in our body were made in the stars of heaven. The universe is literally in us, as we are in the universe. A state of grace is developed when we can maintain our ability to stay in the presence of this awareness.

"I am in the universe.
The universe is in my body
The universe and I are one"
Chunyi Lin, Spring Forest Qigong

Practice Form One:
Simple Standing in Wuji

Place your feet at least shoulder width apart and parallel to each other. Feel rooted into the earth beneath your feet. Bend your knees slightly and feel how bending your knees enables you to relax more deeply. Make sure your knees are bent in the same direction as your toes. Feel the nourishing support of Mother Earth. Take a moment to feel gratitude for the earth, which nourishes our body with food, water and oxygen and sustains our spirit with the beauty of nature.

Find your center of gravity and relax around your axis. Bring your mind's loving attention into your body. Close your eyes or soften them to avoid outer distraction. Relax your tailbone down. Feel your hips relaxing over your two soft strong legs. Feel the pelvic girdle, the basket of bones holding up the trunk of your body. Relax your shoulders over your hips and feel the organs in the trunk of your body settle down and relaxed to do their job. Tuck your chin in, to lengthen the back of your neck. Feel the head lightly lift up as if you were being pulled up to heaven with a silver thread.

Now you can feel yourself dangling from this thread and aligning through your axis with the earth. Open the crown of your head to the big blue sky, the heavenly energy of the cosmos and all the beautiful stars and planets. Know these stars created the elements that make up your body. You are in the universe and the universe is in you. Feel the oneness with all there is.

Feel into your breath. Place your hands over your lower dan tian, usually right hand first, left hand cover, just below the navel. This area is a powerful energy field called the field of elixir. The elbows are forward to open the armpits and allow the lymph system to freely flow and support your immune system. Feel yourself between heaven and earth and take your place as part of humanity. Feel your whole body breathing. When you inhale your belly expands slightly and when you exhale your belly contracts slightly. Feel your breath even through the pores of your skin.

Feel into your center line and soften around your axis. Wait for the shift in energy, the quiet, soft, stillness of the meditation stance. Be present in the state of Wuji, the state of not doing, just being. Feel the fullness of being empty, of doing nothing.

Bring your mind's attention into your body. Release any tight places. Breathe into any painful places whether physical, mental, or emotional. Give those tight and painful places some room for change. Allow the Qi to flow through and harmonize and heal your body mind and spirit. Open to a soft awareness.

Practice

Daily Practice

The commitment to daily practice assures the greatest continuous health benefits, not only physically but mentally and emotionally. The cultivated strength, balance and good health are reflected in a long and happy life. By investing time for Qigong and Tai Chi, you will reap these rewards. The lower dan tien is called the "Qi bank account." Daily practice keeps Qi in the "Sea of Qi reservoir" to be used when you need it.

Each person will find a time that works for them. A regular time is usually best. Some like to practice first thing in the morning when they get up. Grand Master Chen Man Ching suggested doing Qigong and Tai Chi before the morning ablutions. He said this was especially true if you lacked discipline and found days that went by without training. Do it first thing and it's done. Others like a midday reprieve to refresh themselves. Many people in China have group Qigong or Tai Chi available in their workplace at lunch time. There is evidence that with the midday practice, work production is greater in the afternoon. Taking time at the end of the workday is also a good way to transition from work to personal time. With a daily practice, you can return to the solace of the self to center and refresh.

Individual practice can be very familiar and satisfying. It gets to be a habit like brushing your teeth. If you don't do it, you miss it. Practice becomes a friend you have a date with. It's a familiar relationship, yet you can always discover something new.

Group Practice

Standing or moving meditation is often done in cooperation with everyone else when we practice Qigong or Tai Chi in a group. It is best performed outdoors in a natural setting like in a park. Choose a peaceful setting with fresh air and fairly level ground, a place where you can reflect a peaceful fresh energy within.

There are great benefits of practicing in a class with other people. Every person brings their own energy field of Qi to the group and together the whole field becomes denser, wider, and stronger. As Aristotle said, "The whole is greater than the sum of its parts." When individuals are connected together in unity, their combined energy can be used as a greater pool of energy for all to bathe in. This unified field offers more energy than we can access by ourselves. We become one entity connected and united.

Group energy has a motivating factor. Having a regular class offers connections, friendships, and camaraderie. Over the years of practice together we have a sense of being in a family. As in a good family, class can be a place of refuge to relax and restore and feel the support of others.

Finding a Teacher

Over the forty-five years of my practice, I've seen a huge growth in the popularity of Qigong and Tai Chi. Now there are many videos and books on these ancient arts, but you can only learn so much from a book or a video. As I have stated, it is good to have a teacher and a group to practice with. Qigong and Tai Chi are living art forms.

Qigong and Tai Chi classes are held in parks, community centers, senior centers, gyms, hospitals and privately. Every teacher is different. Every group is unique. If you don't like a teacher, learn what you can and be open to finding another teacher who works for you. Every teacher can provide something valuable.

TWO

Out of Nothing
Comes Something

The Great Void created the Tao, the Tao
created yin and yang, the pair of harmonious
energies that continue to create all there is.

The Beginning

Finding my Teacher

After the Country Women's Festival, I looked for a woman teacher. There were very few teachers of Tai Chi in 1975, and the few women I found were too far away for me to attend class. After months of searching, I found an advertisement in the Sonoma Index Tribune for a Tai Chi class right in town. I was encouraged and called the number. A man answered. His voice had an unusual quality. He spoke with what sounded like a fake Chinese accent that put me

28

off. I asked if I could take Tai Chi from him. He seemed tentative like he wasn't interested in taking a new student. Then he laughed and told me to come the next day to the old Junior High School building at 9am to begin my Tai Chi training.

The next morning I walked into the abandoned school that had been converted to a Community Center. At the end of a long hall was a lovely large classroom. It had the original highly polished dark-wood floors which glowed in the morning sun spilling through big windows. The many small paned windows covered the entire length of the southern wall and were open to the street below. But no one was there. The building seemed totally empty, but I found a woman in the office downstairs. She told me she didn't know why there wasn't a class that day and assured me that I was in the right place.

Discouraged I headed home, passing the beautiful Sonoma Plaza with its historic City Hall, green lawns, rose gardens, and children's playground. In the distance I saw a group of people doing some strange movements that I guessed might be the Tai Chi class. I parked my car and wandered over to find a very tall, exotic looking black man wearing a Chinese jacket and a Taoist cap leading the class.

I listened on the edge of the irregular circle of students until he acknowledged me. I asked why he hadn't told me the class was in the park. He replied with a laugh that it was my first lesson. I was to use my psychic powers of intuition to find him. I was a little annoyed by this somewhat flippant answer but signed up to come to the full four days a week of training. He instructed me to call him Sifu Nam Singh. What kind of name is that? I questioned to myself. I thought he must be a Sikh. I wondered how this black man with a Sikh name learned the ancient art of Tai Chi. This man became my root Tai Chi teacher, my beloved Sifu Nam Singh.

Dragon Tiger Mountain Tai Chi Chuan with Sifu Nam Singh

Thursday's class was an evening class from 7:00 to 9:00 PM. Sifu Nam Singh was reviewing the first movements of the Dragon Tiger Mountain long form and having the students repeat the form and move in unison. He reviewed what the class had learned and made personal posture corrections. Then he had us follow him in the performance of the full 108 movements. Even though no one knew what they were doing, we followed him the best we could. We all stumbled around. It was frustrating and yet beautiful.

The form was done very slowly as if we were all moving together underwater. I thought that I should be able to follow easily because it was so slow, but I was often on the wrong foot or had the wrong arm up. It felt awkward and embarrassing, but it was exciting to be a part of everyone moving together. We were in three lines, four abreast. At moments, when everyone came together, the group moved like one animal. We faced forward and then turned to the West moving slowly forward. We'd turn in the air, and flow into what he called "White Crane Stands on one Leg," or some other poetically named posture. He would call out the names of the movements as we imitated his graceful gestures.

As the weeks went by the form became easier and more coherent. At times we became a slow whirl of oneness until we once again came back to where we started for a final bow after a flurry of eight kicks to every direction. Sometimes my legs would ache from keeping a low stance for the twenty minutes it took to do 108 movements and yet I felt exhilarated with some strange satisfaction I'd never felt before.

After the form we took a short break. Then Sifu would show the class the next movement. The class had already been meeting for several weeks when I started. I asked Sifu to please teach me the first five movements so I could catch up. He assigned two of the new students to show me what they'd learned. Then he tested me and them, correcting the teachings I'd been given.

It made me very nervous to be singled out. I wanted to run out of the room, but I got through it. When I got home, I practiced what I'd learned immediately so I could remember how to do the moves correctly and not suffer the embarrassment of exposing my flaws and errors to the other students. Daily practice strengthened my ability. Sometimes I couldn't remember exactly how to flow from one position to the next but when I got it, there was a feeling of surprise, delight, and satisfaction.

Sifu Nam Singh was a harsh teacher. He would push our stamina to the limit. He would have us stand perfectly still with our arms held out in front of us as if we were embracing a big tree. We held 90% of our weight on one foot and 10% on the ball of the other foot placed out in front of our body in what he called "Cat Stance." We would stand for about twenty minutes. I could feel the muscles of my thighs and calves tremble and spasm. I took some comfort in the fact that the guy in front of me in Bermuda shorts was also having spasms. We didn't dare give up or we'd suffer humiliation. If our arms would sag, he'd come over and reposition them to the correct level. Then he'd sharply pat our shoulders and command, "Relax!" It was tough and about half of the class quit after a few weeks. Then he'd say, "Good! Now we got rid of the riff raff and have serious practitioners that don't waste my time."

In some sessions we wouldn't do the Tai Chi form at all. He would just have us do the standing practice and then we'd walk around the edges of the room in a line. We would fill the empty space in front of us, then fill another empty space as we moved forward with each step. We moved slowly in coordination with our breath all the way around the big room for about half an hour or more.

Sometimes I'd be bored and irritable. Sometimes I'd fall into a trance-like state. Sometimes I'd get insight on true patience. Walking in a line also taught us to be aware of the person in front of us. If we moved too fast, we'd be stepping on their heels, so we learned to pace ourselves with others, not too fast and not too slow.

Sifu shared many different practices. We never knew what he'd have up his sleeves. And his costumes varied almost as much as his practices. Sometimes he came in ornate full-length robes or classic Tai Chi uniforms. He often wore various turbans and other exotic looking hats. Sometimes he would show up in casual western clothes like Bermuda shorts and a shirt with sandals as if he'd just come back from the beach.

Nam Singh was mysterious, strict, and yet jovial. He loved to laugh. He had smooth brown skin, big flashing brown eyes, and he sported a small beard or goatee. His Tai Chi form was exquisite, a seamless floating body of energy. His beautiful hands the final expression of the movement that seemed to come from the core of the earth, yet light as a feather. There was no effort in his movements. He was a being of continuous harmony and grace. It wasn't only when he did the form, but his every movement was even, thoughtful, and effortless. Watching him cook was as satisfying as watching a classic ballet. One movement followed the next without anxiety. He was smooth and powerful. I adored him. I mimicked him to try to capture in myself that ease of continuous flow.

There was so much to learn. It was challenging for me to attain the muscle strength for slow, continuous flow with flexibility and balance. My mind was also challenged in remembering the many sequences in the form. Sometimes I was discouraged but over time I felt more confident. I became captivated by the adventure of learning Tai Chi. I loved the poetry of the names of its movements, learning about its long history, and the philosophy behind the practice. Like acupuncture, Qigong and Tai Chi Chuan are part of Traditional Chinese Medicine. For me this study opened up a rich and wonderful world.

Writing, Lineage, Ritual

The spelling that we know as Tai Chi Chuan is from the Wade Gilles translation. The proper spelling is taijiquan, which is the modern Pinyin translation.

In Pinyin, Tai translates as great. The ji is translated as pole or extreme, so taiji represents perfect balance and harmony with duality, but the word or character for Chi or Qi is absent. However, Qi is the energy of the universe that is made of yin/yang. It is the energy we cultivate in our practice. So, you can see my spelling is a little mixed, as with many westerners at this time. We keep the Tai Chi Chuan as the translation for the continuous slow-moving forms that are now practiced around the world. However, we recognize the new spelling of Qigong for the shorter health exercises of TCM that have become more popular in the last twenty years.

Forty years ago, Qigong was spelled Chi Kung or Chi Gung. It is part of what makes China so mysterious. The Pinyin system strains our ability to pronounce or even recognize Chinese words. It seems they took the most difficult English letters of x, z and q and put them in everything. They break the English rules of always placing a "u" after "q" which takes a bit of getting used to. The challenge is worth the effort.

Learning to read the Chinese characters is even more rewarding, since they were standardized over 2000 years ago, yet still retain their pictographic essence. People can still read ancient scripts, whereas in the west our calligraphy has changed so much our grandchildren can't even read our cursive.

The brush strokes of Chinese calligraphy depict simple lines that symbolize the object they represent. The characters have been simplified through thousands of years but still retain some of the pictographic characteristics.

In China, there are many dialects and people from different provinces that may sound different from each other. The written words look the same, they are just pronounced differently. When I was in Shanghai, the business capital of China, people from different districts could not understand each other. They would try to speak in Mandarin and if that didn't work, they would try English. Many people in China learn English and Mandarin, which is the official standard spoken language of China. It is called the speech of the officials.

Chinese culture is one of the oldest living cultures on earth. Their written language began with the Shang Dynasty and their oracle bones. The ancient scripts, found on bones and tortoise shells, have evolved into today's Chinese characters. Beautiful calligraphy painted with brush and ink is an art form. Calligraphy is one of the five masteries of the scholar/sage.

My Sifu Nam Singh said that it is traditional for teachers to practice painting, sculpture and poetry as well as martial arts. His Grand Master Chen Man Ching, or sometimes spelled Jan Man Ching, is recognized for his mastery of calligraphy as well as his mastery of Tai Chi. In Chinese martial arts masters keep a balance between art and war. When I was sculpting and practicing Tai Chi, I felt lucky to be in tune with this custom.

The Tao Created the Tai Chi

Where there is movement there is Yin and Yang

"There is a chaotic thing, born before heaven and earth. So silent. So empty, unique and unchanging. Circling endlessly, it could be called the Mother of All Things Under Heaven. I do not know its name. I reluctantly call it Tao, and if forced to do so, would describe it as great."
Chapter 25, Tao te Ching, by
Lao Tzu, about 500 BC

Tai Chi, like Traditional Chinese Medicine, is based on the ancient philosophy of Taoism or Daoism which is translated as The Way. It is a study of being in harmony with nature. The Taoists describe the universe coming into being from nothing. In Tai Chi philosophy it is said, "out of nothing came something." This is called the great Tao or The Way. The Way is the order of the universe and its creation. It's how things work.

> **Tao produced the natural order, which gives rise to the constant changes made by the play of yin and yang.**

We can describe the qualities of nature in the terms of yin and yang. For instance, yin's quality is cold, heavy, dark and sinks; whereas yang is hot, light, and rises. Fire is yang as heat rises. Water is yin as it sinks down into the earth. Nature is a balance of yin and yang. It gives and receives in ever flowing cycles. Seeds grow into plants and plants produce more seeds. Life reproduces itself through the action of yin and yang. Youth is flexible, resilient, and active. The old get stiff, brittle and die. These actions are natural and represent the harmony of Tao.

I am astounded that modern science and ancient Taoist's teachings relate so closely. Physicists tell us our universe began about fourteen billion years ago from a dense, hot point of singularity. They call it "The Big Bang." Everything in our immense Cosmos, which is larger than we can conceive, came from a tiny point that is still unknowable.

After the Big Bang, tiny particles bound together to form hydrogen and helium. As time went on, young stars formed when clouds of gas and dust gathered under the effect of gravity, heating up as they became denser. At the stars' cores, bathed in temperatures of over 10 million degrees centigrade, hydrogen created the atom of helium and the helium nuclei fused to form heavier elements.

Everything is made of elements. Elements are pure substance made of atoms that are all the same type. At present, 116 elements are known, and about 90 of these occur naturally. If you look at the periodic chart from your high school science class, you find lists of all the elements in neat rows and columns. Hydrogen is on the far left of the periodic chart with 1 proton, 1 neutron and 1 electron. Helium is on the far right with 2 protons, 2 neutrons and 2 electrons.

Helium is created by two hydrogen atoms. Hydrogen accounts for about three quarters of the atoms in the universe and Helium makes up the other quarter. A remaining 4% make up the heavier atoms in the universe.

If we consider that yin and yang made up everything in the universe, we can think of hydrogen as yin, open and receptive and helium as yang, closed and complete in itself. The hydrogen atom is eager to find something to fill the empty space and two hydrogen atoms connect easily with one oxygen atom to make H_2O or water. Helium is a noble gas. Noble gases do not combine with other atoms.

We are Stardust

In Qigong practice we say, "We are in the universe and the universe is in us." In the scientific understanding this is literally true. As the cloud of cosmic dust and gases from the Big Bang cooled, stars formed, and these then grouped together forming galaxies. Nuclear reactions in the stars and in huge stellar explosions created the elements found in nature. Stars explode at the end of their lives; the resulting high energy environment enables the creation of some of the heavier elements including iron, nickel, and gold. The explosions disperse the elements they create across the universe. The stardust scatters making the planets, including our Earth, and us.

> **We are in the universe,
> and the universe is in us.**

The sun is yang because it is characterized by light and warmth. From our perspective it appears to move across the sky. The earth is considered yin because of gravity and its cold, solid nature. Yin night is graced by the yin moon. She is called the "The Queen of the Night" as she moves the yin waters which are the womb of life.

The Harmonious Qi, Yin-Yang Energy

Practitioners of Chinese Traditional Medicine believe Qigong practice balances yin-yang energy in many ways. At the beginning of our practice, we align with the yin Earth and the yang Heaven. The play of yin-yang energy is the basis for Tai Chi and Qi gong.

The Tao produces the pulsating forces of yin (off) and yang (on). Qi is energy and always made of yin and yang. Energy is frequency and vibration that move atomic particles and form the elements of our universe. The crest is yang, the trough is yin. Yin-yang are always in harmony. They are the opposing forces of nature, polar opposites. There is no yin without yang. You can't have an up without a down, or a back without a front, or in without out. Yin-yang energy is in constant motion as yin flows into yang and yang becomes yin. It is relative. Your right is on my left. The brush when it is at rest on the table is yin. It is yang when you fill it with ink and use it. The paper is yin when it is blank, and yang when it projects the image of your creation.

In Tai Chi the sinking force of yin gathers the active uprooting ability of yang. Sink low to go high. Center in to spiral out. The body remains relaxed and centered around its axis. The spiraling power of yang force emerges from its center. The tighter a spring winds, the stronger the power it releases. In the Tai Chi form when you take a step, the moving foot is yang. When you shift your weight onto the foot, it becomes yin. The full becomes empty and the empty full.

The symbol for yin-yang is called the Tai Chi. It depicts two fish swimming within a circle of unity. One fish changes into the other as the two fish swim in constant motion. There is a little yin in the yang, and a little yang in the yin. Stillness becomes movement and movement becomes stillness. The empty becomes full and what is full returns to emptiness.

From the great void of Wuji came Tai Chi.
Tai Chi is made up of energy pulsating
in yin-yang frequency.

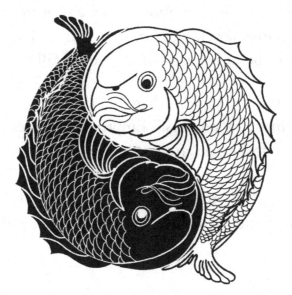

Yin Yang Fish by Margaret Emerson

In doing the Tai Chi form the principles of yin and yang become embodied. Tai Chi is a "moving meditation." It begins from a standing position of equal weight cultivating the yin qualities of stillness and emptiness. The practitioner brings their attention to their breath. The breath is a yin inhale and a yang exhale.

From the emptiness of Wuji and Simple Standing, the deep inhale breath creates a propensity for the arms to raise which is yang force, and for the body to settle and sink which is yin force. The sinking down and shifting the weight to the right foot allows the empty left foot to rise and take a step to the yin left. It is an empty step with no weight. The body weight shifts and moves in lightness, with our exhale, which is yang energy. The left foot slowly fills, becoming yin and solid. Yin becomes yang, yang returns to yin in flowing motion as we continue the form. When we move far enough to the right, we have to move to the left to be in balance, or we would fall over.

We learn the principle, "there is stillness in movement and movement in stillness." Emptiness purifies the space so that the movements are not driven by muscle strength. Coordinated with our breath, the natural Qi flows from one movement to the next. The act of emptying clears away tension and stress. We "empty the cup to fill it," says Lao Tzu.

Qi is Energy

When Qi condenses it forms matter, when
it disperses it becomes energy.

Chang Tsai says:

"When Qi condenses, its visibility becomes apparent,
so that there are then the shapes of individual things.
When it disperses its visibility is no longer
apparent and there are no shapes.
At the time of its condensation
can one say otherwise then that this is but temporary?
But at the time of its dispersing
can one hastily say that it is then non-existent?"

We live in fields of energy. Each field is connected and interacting with other fields. Fields enfold into themselves and into other fields in an endless process of creation and destruction.

Elisabeth Rochat de la Vallee, an expert on Chinese characters and philosophy, writes, "Qi was originally thought of as wind, a wind of heaven, penetrating the earth." Eventually Qi was linked to what brought life into being. "Qi is neither substance or spirit, yet it manifests through all forms and forces." The form is yin, the force is yang.

> **"Qi is neither substance nor spirit yet it manifests though all forms and forces."**

Taoism and Nature

Sifu told us the first symbol of yin and yang was a mountain with a dark and a light side. The north side is dark and cold and considered yin. The light, warm, sunny south side is yang. Knowing where and when to plant in the agrarian culture of ancient China was essential for an abundant harvest.

The Chinese have been studying the sky for thousands of years. The Imperial court had astronomers and mathematicians whose chief ranked as a Minister of State and annually submitted his work to the Emperor for approval. When the Sovereign pronounced it good, copies of the new almanac were distributed to the highest officials of the Empire. The almanacs were received with Imperial honors. They were carried to their destinations in sedan chairs, placed on pedestals, and greeted with prostrations and a salute of guns on New Year's Day. The Book of Records contains notices given by the Perfect Emperor Yao in 2254 BCE to his astronomers commanding them to ascertain the solstices and equinoxes so the farmer might know when to plant.

Following lunar cycles, the Chinese created their calendar. The moon, according to the Chinese, belongs to the Earth. The lunar calendar has Ten Heavenly Stems which correlate to the Five Elements and Twelve Earthly Branches, which are associated with the twelve animals of the Chinese zodiac.

The creation of the calendar is told in a charming story of a great race. The God of Heaven, Yu Huang or Yu Di, is known as The Jade Emperor. It is told that he called the animals to run a race to decide the order of the Chinese zodiac. Each position in the Chinese zodiac represents twelve years in a sixty-year cycle.

The race starts with the confused Tiger who asks the Rat directions to the Jade Emperor. The Rat lies to the Tiger to divert him and therefore the cat has been enemies with the rat ever since. The Rat scurries along until he reaches the river which he cannot cross. He persuades the Ox to take him across on his horns. Having crossed the great river, the Rat jumps down and takes his place as first.

Many people cringe when they hear that a rat is included in the pantheon of animals. But consider the importance of this little character. In the last great extinction, when the asteroid hit the Yucatan 65 million years ago, most of life on the planet perished. The only mammal to survive was a creature very like the rat. So perhaps he deserves the honor of being in first place.

> *In Qigong and Tai Chi, we practice the awareness of Qi and its movement. We feel Qi move through us, guide our actions, enter and exit our body, surround us and connect us to Qi fields of heaven, earth, and life around us.*

Practice Two:
The Bow

I like to start my Qigong class in a circle so we can feel the energy of the group. The energy of each person in the class connects to every other person and makes what we call a Qi field. Often this energy is very strong. The whole is more than the sum of its parts. We combine our energy and all benefit from sharing the loving light of Qi.

Qigong practice starts with Wuji Standing which connects us to our core of stillness. In Simple Standing we focus to align with the powers of earth and heaven. Finally, we bring our attention to our breath and the power of our own humanity. To conclude the Standing the leader says, "Kuan Li!" The practitioners respond, "Kuan Li!"

Kuan Li

Kuan Li is a salute that means, "merciful behavior." It is a good reminder as we start our practice to be kind to ourselves, to others and to nature itself. Kuan means compassionate contemplation. Li means natural behavior. The Chinese see Li in the grain or pattern of wood or jade. The swirls and knots in the wood are its natural behavior, the way it grows through its own DNA. Our natural Li is what makes us unique through our ancestry, physical appearance and propensities. When we bow, we pay respect and honor who we truly are; we also respect others in the group and their uniqueness; finally we respect nature itself and seek through understanding to be in harmony with Her.

Chain Link of Grace

We bring our feet together and raise our hands up from our sides gathering energy from earth and heaven. With our hands over our head, we make a fist with our right hand and cover it with our left. This is a hand position, a mudra, called the Chain Link of Grace.

The mudra of the Chain Link of Grace is made up of the Boxer and the Scholar. The right hand forms a closed fist which is yang action and the symbol of the boxer. The left hand is yin and symbolizes the scholar. It is open and represents a book and our own inner teacher, the intuition we find within. The right side of the body is usually considered yang. The masculine quality of action and movement is yang. The still feminine qualities are yin. Outside is yang. Inside is yin. Full is yang. Empty is yin. The mind is yang. The body is yin.

The Chain Link of Grace drifts down the center of the body in acknowledgement of all three dan tiens or energy centers. The upper dan tien is in the head, the middle is in the chest and heart, and the lower dan tien is just below the navel. The dan tiens are energy centers called "fields of elixir." They are also called the Three Fields of Cinnabar and they are alchemical areas of the body that can change disharmony into harmony.

The Chain Link of Grace hand mudra drops through the body like a pearl dropping through oil. It moves through the three dan tiens to the base where the hands naturally turn with the thumbs on top. The shoulders are relaxed. The body bends forward at the hips while keeping the back straight. The eyes connect with the others in the circle, or they look towards the horizon.

The folded hands salute three times in honoring mind, body and spirit. The fist drops out and comes up around the left-hand. The hands circle around each other as the body straightens up to standing in alignment. The left foot steps out to bring the feet shoulder width apart and parallel. The palms drift down to the sides as the body weight sinks down into the earth. The palms face back, opening the arm pits to allow the lymph system to freely flow.

In stillness the belly fills with the inhale and contracts with the exhale. With the inhale the arms rise, with the exhale the arms sink. The whole body is breathing.

The bow can used to start or end any form, whether in a group or alone. It gives a sense of entering or exiting a Qi field. It prepares us for a change like walking through a doorway or threshold. The bow creates an awareness of something being set aside as special and acknowledged.

Practice Three: Harmonize with the Qi

You may want to set an intention. I particularly like this one: "I work for a healthy body, a healthy community and a healthy earth."

With this simple practice we can heal our body and allow new ideas and new possibilities to arise. As we relax and refresh ourselves, we let go of old patterns and habits.

Place your feet about shoulder width apart. Open your palms forward keeping your shoulders relaxed. Let go of preconceptions and distractions, just be fresh and present with an awareness of the environment that surrounds you.

In this intentional peaceful state, focus your attention inside. Pay attention to your breath. Allow your body to relax and breathe into every cell. Say the affirmation, "I breath the pure Qi of the universe into every cell of my body." Feel the healing harmonizing power of Qi. Feel the loving light renew and rejuvenate your whole being.

Practice Four:
Filling and Emptying

From the meditative posture in Practice Three, place your hands on your belly just below your navel, right hand against your belly, left hand covering the right. Shift your weight onto your right foot. Feel the weight fill the right side of your body. Stay upright and relaxed. You may close or soften your eyes to find your balance point. Pick up your left heel without moving any other part of your body to test that your weight is fully on the right foot. Feel the emptiness of your left foot. Begin to move your center over to fill the left foot and empty the right foot. Feel as if you were filling a glass of water and then emptying the glass. When the left is full, lift the right heel and lower it without any movement in your shoulders or hips. Feel which foot is empty and which is full as you move your center line slowly back and forth, intentionally filling one as you empty the other. Inhale into center and exhale as you shift your weight. When the foot has weight, it is called solid. When it has no weight, it is called empty. Continue this practice moving side to side for about five minutes or thirty-two breaths.

Practice Five:
Simple Taoist Walking

You can use the same principle of filling and emptying as you walk forward slowly. Place the empty foot in front of you. Slowly and evenly move your weight to fill it; Then pick up the empty back foot softly placing it in front of you. Keep your shoulders relaxed over your hips throughout the movements. As you continue this walking practice focus on how yin turns to yang and yang turns to yin, how empty becomes full and full becomes empty.

THREE

Energy Fields, The Three Powers, The Three Treasures

Class with Sifu

One late summer day in the upper room of the old schoolhouse where our Tai Chi class was held, Sifu Nam Singh offered us something unusual. Sifu had us lie on our backs on the old wood floor in a big circle. It was a pleasant morning. The sun came through the small paned windows making little square shadows on the polished floor. There were about twelve of us maneuvering to find floor space with arm's distance between each of us. I placed my scarf under my head for a cushion against the hard floor and got comfortable. Sifu said we were going to do a sound meditation. We settled down and waited.

The beginning of the meditation was silent. We were all listening. Then Sifu started laughing, and we all started laughing. We laughed until we couldn't laugh anymore. I could feel the tears roll down my cheeks, my stomach hurt and the muscles in my face were tired of laughing. The laugher subsided and there would be a silent space, but then someone would let out a snicker and laughter would overtake us. We couldn't stop even when we tried.

Finally, after a minute or two of silence, I started hearing a faint sound. I didn't know where it was coming from or what it was. It was a soft sound that vibrated throughout the room. The enchanting hum was a continuous monotone that took me far away.

I found my mind riding on the sound. Then the hum changed to other tones and I was swept away in waves drifting through intricate layers of vibration and frequency.

I felt my spirit leap out of my body. Suddenly, I was flying across a desert. A hot wind lifted me as I zoomed over ochre colored sands. I felt the warmth of the desert radiating up into me. Then I felt a chill come over me. I was flying over mountain tops along a ridgeline, darting along cliffs that dropped into a churning sea of dark blue. I felt I could go anywhere in the world. I was gliding over the surface of the earth. Hot wet tears of joy ran down the sides of my cheeks and into my hair and ears.

This was one of the most memorable events in my life. It was an out-of-body experience. After this experience I felt I knew what was meant by astral travel.

The finale was a gong crescendo, becoming so intense it filled the room with an overpowering crashing sound. The sound shocked me back into my body. I felt transformed. I had crossed a threshold of knowledge, but I couldn't really say what I had learned. It was beyond words. The room returned to silence.

We just lay there assimilating the strange and wonderful experience. Slowly we began sitting up, coming to in our various ways, speechless and grateful. Years later Sifu gifted me the precious gong, though it has never sounded so magical as the day he gave us the sound healing.

Three Powers

Heaven, Earth and Humanity are the Three Powers which are called San Tsai. Connecting to these powers gives us access to increased vitality, mental awareness and spiritual insight. We are not here to struggle alone, as we try to maintain ourselves. We can turn to the gifts freely given by the power of earth, the power of heaven, and the power of our breath and body.

The Three Powers are fundamental to any Qigong practice. Alignment and connection of our body to Earth and Heaven softens and opens us. When we are in alignment, we get the sense we are dangling from heaven while being rooted in earth. Being rooted allows us to surrender to earth's gravity and gives us a feeling of relaxation.

> # Alignment and connection of our body to Earth and Heaven softens and opens us.

The Qigong practitioner learns to balance and harmonize these powers for good health, healing, and grace. When I go to my practice place and connect to the Three Powers, I feel a sense of grace moving through me physically and spiritually. When I am connected to the Three Powers it feels as if my forms are without effort. I'm not doing them; they are doing me.

The Power of Earth gives us material form. We are part of the body of this living planet Earth. Earth is like the trunk of a tree and we are Her branches. Her elements and microorganisms live within our body. Earth gives us the power to inherit and reproduce. Earth gives us the ability to express love in all its forms, whether it's enjoying sexuality, hugging our friends and children, writing a poem or singing a love song. Earth nourishes our body by providing food, water, and the air we breathe. She restores our spirit with Her beauty.

Heavenly Qi is the force in the universe which created everything that exists from the beginning of time. The power of Heaven is the expansive energy. Science holds that the Cosmos has been expanding ever since the Big Bang. We feel the power of Heaven in the big blue sky and in the light of the life-giving sun. The power of heaven establishes time, the laws of nature, cause and effect. Heavenly Qi gives us creative energy, curiosity, and imagination. When we are aware of our connection and inter-dependence, we are in touch with the power of Heaven.

Finally, we feel the power of humanity when we breathe into our body. Our energy and our bodily form are our link between heaven and earth. When we feel a unity with heaven and earth energies, we realize that life is more than just the isolation of our small self. We feel our connection with all of humanity, and we are in touch with the magnificent mystery of life on this planet.

The Tai Chi Circle

When I go to my Tai Chi circle to practice, I feel a sense of excitement. I walk onto the area of green grass in my back yard where I teach my Saturday class. A redwood and a large oak tree in the south shade half the lawn and I can choose to be in sun or shade. In the northwest corner a giant silver maple spreads its majestic branches to the sky. Acorn woodpeckers make nests in the knot holes. I'd count five or six birds here for several years.

Last year, I think the grey squirrel that recently moved in may have destroyed their nest. I missed their chattering back and forth to each other. I was delighted to find that this year honeybees have taken over the knot hole and I pray for their well-being. Everything changes, I remind myself as I stand in the middle of this well-loved field facing black bamboo and a simple sculpture designating true north.

My Tai Chi circle is a safe place for me to honor Mother Earth and Father Sky. I feel myself as their child, being held in their embrace. I am grounded like the trees, present and still, surrounded by the mystery of time-space in the eternal now. The energy is expansive, positive and open. My body feels like it's subtly glowing, with a radiant energy.

I check-in with how I am. My breath guides me as I find my balanced center. I begin moving. I concentrate and feel my movements becoming smooth and steady. I feel the air is thick as water. The Qi moves out from my center as I execute the movements. The space itself has a presence to it. Cutting through, with intentional action, my path meets me as I step into a new direction, placing my foot lightly on the earth.

As I gather and expand, my mind is listening to my body breathe. As I remember the sequence of the movements, my body is listening to my mind. I delight in their poetic names: Pressing Heaven Pressing Earth; The Clouds Touch the Mountain Tops; Reach for the North Star. There is a continuity in the tempo, and a stillness at my center, like the eye of a hurricane. I move this soft center of balance though all the patterns and intricacies of changing direction, weaving the web of protective Qi. Working my limbs, testing my balance, I listen to my breath and remember where I am in the 108 possibilities of change.

This simple act of Tai Chi refreshes my senses, my attitude, and my whole body. I am renewed and happy. I return to a place of power where my ability to choose how I use my energy is clear.

The power of humanity is the power to choose. We are continually giving and receiving Qi. We experience our power of choice as we face each moment in creation. The power of chuan, which is taking responsibility for our self, is expressed by doing the best we can with what we've got. Practice gives us the clarity we need to make healthy choices.

"We are what we repeatedly do; excellence,
then, is not an act but a habit." Aristotle

Through practice we become less distracted. We are fully engaged in the moment. As we do our forms, we become aware of our individuality and our connection to all of humanity. By connecting to Heaven and Earth, we become grounded and more loving. Our intellect, emotions, and empathy act together and then we can act with integrity.

Through the practice of Wuji, we cultivate
The Three Powers of Earth, Heaven, and Humanity.

Practice Six:
Three Powers Practice

In this Qigong practice we connect to the power of earth's gravity. Gravity is the root of our balance. When we find the center line of alignment, we can surrender to Mother Earth. We can relax. We let the earth support our weight. Using the Power of Earth, we completely relax our body around the centerline axis.

Place your feet shoulder width apart and parallel. Bend your knees and sink down, working with gravity to soften your body. Feel the balanced connection with earth energy. The dark, cool, moist, nurturing energy of mother earth is the yin quality of condensing Qi. The one point of gravity establishes your centerline. Feel your gratitude for earth which sustains and nourishes you with her abundance. Feel the roots of your energetic tree, reaching down into the earth. Experience the stillness of the yin energy.

When we are in balance with the yin softness,
there is no strain on any part of the body.
We are centered and relaxed and open to
the internal movement of yang.

Your head lightly lifts up toward heaven as if were being pulled up by a silver thread. You feel as if you are dangling from heaven, like a plum bob, in line with gravity. Feel the alignment of heaven and earth meeting through your centerline and connecting at the lower dan tien, just below your naval.

Open the crown of your head and feel as if your head touches the big blue sky. Open to the radiant energy of the cosmos and of the expanding universe. Feel the primal original Qi of creation, the Yuan Qi. Feel into the loving, peaceful, radiant Power of Heaven, the loving light.

Finally, bring your mind's attention into the third power, the Power of Breath, your body, and your humanity. Place your attention on the internal sensations of your breath. Explore the nature of your inhale and your exhale. Ask yourself, "Is my breath deep or shallow?" Experience how your whole body is involved in your breathing. Find the movement in the stillness of your breath. Find the stillness in the movement of your breath. Feel your whole body breathing in alignment between heaven and earth.

You may enjoy using this simple reminder of alignment with the Three Powers:

Feet stand on earth
Head touches sky
Whole body breathing

Torus Field of Energy

The torus is a donut shape of moving, spiraling, protective energy that surrounds our body, our cells, the earth itself, and our Milky Way galaxy. The torus is the shape of electromagnetic energy. We can understand our energy body in both scientific and mystical terms. It can be understood scientifically as an electromagnetic field. A torus shaped field of electromagnetic energy surrounds our body, our own atmosphere of Qi.

Electro-magnetism is created by positive and negative energy poles and light. EM radiation is a form of energy that is all around us and takes many forms, such as radio waves, microwaves, X-rays and gamma rays. Sunlight is also a form of EM energy; however visible light is only a small portion of the EM spectrum. The EM spectrum contains a broad range of electromagnetic wavelengths.

The energy surrounding living bodies has been measured by science through Kirlian photography, which has revealed a ghostly aura body of a whole leaf even after part of it had been torn away. The leaf's energy body left an imprint of the whole intact leaf.

There are many human energy fields. These include the physically measurable electromagnetic and magnetic fields generated by all living cells, tissues, organs and the body as a whole. There are also biofields, subtle fields emanating from these pulsing units of life. Biofields are characterized as physical fields that regulate the human body. Emotional fields regulate emotional states. Mental fields process ideas, thoughts and beliefs. The astral field is thought of as a nexus between the physical and spiritual realms.

The way I see it, everything has an energy field. There are fields within fields, from the cosmic consciousness right down to the quantum level. Our human energy field that is connected to earth and sky is constantly processing the energy fields that we meet through conscious and unconscious connections. To get along well, we can simply connect to the guidance of our heart.

The powerful heart has its own torus field. The company, HeartMath, has measured the torus field surrounding the heart. It shows that the energy field of the heart extends several feet from our body. When we strengthen this field by connecting to our center and receiving the natural love of the heart, we make loving connections and decisions which protect us from emotional stress that can lead to physical illness.

Mystical Energy Fields

Ancient religious practices around the world understand energy fields and the power of the spirit. Many of these practices acknowledge an etheric energy field around the human body called an aura. The Hindus in ancient India see the aura as containing seven chakras each with its own specific energy field. Christians see a halo of light signifying greater spiritual enlightenment. The disciples of Jesus at the Pentecost saw what seemed to be tongues of fire that separated and a tongue of fire rested on each of their heads. This was known by the Christians as the baptism by fire. It was an enlightenment that gave them power to prophesy and heal.

The energy body that surrounds you is like a second skin. This subtle energy body protects and shields our energy system just as physical skin protects our inner organs. Subtle bodies, energy bodies and luminous radiation surround us. Everything we do or think, the forcefields of the planet and frequencies such as radio waves that penetrate us, may affect our aura. Our aura reflects our mental, emotional, physical, and spiritual states. You may know depressed people who seem to be in a dark cloud. We can often feel the positive and negative energy of others and feel its effect on our own energy.

Paracelsus, a Swiss doctor from the German Renaissance who lived 500 years ago, said, "The vital force is not enclosed in man but radiates within and around him like a luminous sphere. It may poison the essence of life and create disease, or it may purify and restore health."

Qigong and Tai Chi support and strengthen our torus field. Sifu said that when we engage our centerline and move our arms, we are spinning a web of energy around our body like cotton candy. The paper cone at the center is wrapped in continuous threads of soft cotton candy like a pink cloud. This wrapping of energy protects our body from disease and air-borne pathogens according to Qigong masters.

When our feet are grounded into the earth, and we are aligned with the loving light of heaven, a free-flowing positive energy is created that moves through and around our body. The conscious use of the Three Powers amplifies this energy.

Kinds of Energy

Yin/Yang energy

The pulsing nature of positive and negative energy creates everything in our physical world. In our universe, matter and energy are made of pairs of opposites: up and down, off and on, energy and matter, force and form.

Skilled acupuncturists are familiar with the subtleties of how Qi works in the body. They describe Qi in terms of yin and yang energy. Qi energy is made of yin and yang, negative and positive energy.

Some examples of Yin and Yang
Qi used by acupuncture:
There is internal qi, and external qi.
There is water qi, and fire qi.
There is stale qi, and fresh qi.

The principle work of the Qigong practitioner and the acupuncturist is to balance the yin and yang energies and their flow throughout the body. Acupuncturists work with specific Qi points where the Qi is close to the surface of the skin. These points are found along the meridians of the body. The acupuncturist places needles at specific points to help Qi flow and harmonize the body and its organs.

The Nei Jing, or Inner Canon, is the oldest book of Traditional Chinese Medicine. It was written over 2000 years ago. It says: "The Meridians move Qi and Blood, regulate Yin and Yang, moisten the tendons and bones, and benefit the joints."

Meridian Qi runs through our bodies along invisible pathways called channels or meridians. The meridians pass through numerous acupuncture points with interesting names like Celestial Pillar on the Governing Vessel, Ultimate Spring on Heart 1, Abundant Prosperity at Stomach 40. Many people go to acupuncturists for a tune-up, especially when seasons change, a time when according to TCM illness can enter the system.

Other Types of Qi

Prenatal Qi is the mysterious primordial energy and cosmic consciousness we have before birth. Prenatal Qi is sometimes called Inherited Qi or Prenatal jing Qi. It is described as vital energy. We are individual aspects of spirit becoming manifested existence at conception. We are given life by the DNA of our ancestors and the primordial energy of cosmic consciousness. Taoists believe the human spirit doesn't die but returns to "our pure nature" when it leaves the body.

Postnatal Qi is formed after birth and comes from the earthly sources of food, water, air and herbs. It is understood that we are given a certain amount of vital energy at birth, our Prenatal Qi. After birth we have Postnatal Qi which we can destroy or protect, depending on our lifestyle and environment. Qigong helps cultivate our Postnatal Qi.

> # Qi, Jing, and Shen are thought of as air, water and fire energy respectively.

The Three Treasures

The three major classifications of Qi manifested in the body are called the Three Treasures or San Bao. They are Qi, Jing, and Shen. There are differences of opinion in the how these types relate to each other. I choose to think of the Three Treasures in this way: the Primal Qi creates the other two forms of Shen and Jing. Qi, Jing and Shen are thought of as air, water and fire energy respectively. Qi is breath. Jing is associated with water and the kidneys. Shen is the fire and light that lives in our heart and mind.

Qi manifests as our breath, as the treasure between heaven and earth imbuing our life from the first to the last breath we take. Our breath determines our life span. Qi breath is also called life force energy. The breath energy within us animates the Shen and Jing.

Primal Qi or Yuan Qi is a vital pulsating force that makes up everything in the cosmos. The personal Shen that lives in our heart and mind is reflected in the larger Heavenly Shen that is cosmic consciousness.

Yuan Qi and DNA

Yuan Qi is the primordial energy we receive at birth. It is the energy of the universe which finds expression in each individual.

"This prenatal spirit is the primordial 'Mind of Tao' which permeates the universe and endows every sentient being with the original light of awareness. Immortal, immaterial and luminous, primordial spirit is the infinite ocean of consciousness from which the eternal spirit of each individual springs. As the transcendent mind of the universe, primordial spirit is the source of wisdom compassion and all spiritual virtue, the guiding light that governs the powers of creation, the master architect of every atom and molecule, star and planet in the ever-expanding temple of the manifest universe." Daniel Reid. A Complete Guide to Chi Gung, Shambala Press, Boston, 2000.

> **Yuan Qi is the Primordial Qi of the universe.**

Yuan Qi is programmed for survival and change. The creative energy of the active yang force moves, creates, and adapts for the survival of its yin material host. Yin is form, and yang is force.

Yuan Qi is infused into our inherited Jing energy. Through Qigong practice we protect, conserve, and enhance our Jing energy. Jing is the consolidation of Qi into solid form. It is a yin energy associated with water. It is the post-natal Qi as described earlier. Post-natal Qi is formed after birth and supported by the earthly sources of food, water, air, and herbs. In Chinese Traditional Medicine the Jing is stored in the Ming Men, the Gate of Life, which is associated with the kidneys and sexuality. The kidney meridian moves from the Bubbling Spring at the bottom of the feet, up the inside of the legs, through the genitals, and up through the kidneys and Ming men. The Ming Men is thought to be where we enter the earth plane.

We are given a certain amount of Jing at birth which we can destroy or protect depending on our lifestyle, environment, and the cultivation of post-natal Qi through diet and exercise. When we use up our Jing energy we die. We deplete our vital essence through overwork, poor diet, and other bodily abuses until we become ill or injured. This is when most people seek to change their ways if they want to restore their good health.

According to Traditional Chinese Medicine, we inherit Jing from our ancestors. The essence of Jing was often translated as semen. The conservation of semen was a Qigong practice to lengthen one's life and good health. I wondered what this had to do with me as a woman. During the patriarchy, when the role of women and the egg was diminished, the sperm was given all the credit for regeneration. Jing is the energy that creates form as our material body. It is the action of the semen and the egg that gives us our inherited propensities.

Jing is thought to be created from the prenatal consciousness of Shen and the force of Qi through the action of our ancestral essence, which we think of as DNA. We are born with predilections for our health through the DNA which we received from both our parents. If long life runs in the family, we will likely have a long life. We are also likely to suffer the illnesses of our ancestors. We are intrinsically connected to all life through the DNA molecule. All known forms of life are based on the same fundamental biochemical organization. Genetic information is encoded in the DNA. The genetic code where DNA information is translated into amino acids is nearly identical for all known life forms including bacteria, single celled microorganisms, animals, and plants. All sexually reproducing organisms are likely derived from a single-celled common ancestor.

The third Treasure, Shen, is the spiritual Qi. The Shen is infused with the "loving light" and lives in our heart and mind. It is referred to as the Immortal Spirit, sometimes called the Eternal or the Deathless. It is our own individual evolving consciousness, which is unique and yet part of the Universal Consciousness. The Shen is the Knower, our true self. It is an energy which is beyond the body yet within the body. Shen is beyond the thinking mind and our emotions. It is an energy linked to eternity and universal consciousness. Through this place at the center of our being we can develop trust and confidence. We train our heart as we gain in understanding. When we are in tune with our Shen, we know love works as a transformative force in our life.

Connecting to Shen requires a state of listening and softening. We have to have the willingness to open our heart. It is like being in the deep humble presence we feel when we pray. Loving Light is a quality of Shen. Shen is the center of our being and serves as a guide to our true self. This loving light shines into our soul and releases our fears, our anger, our worries, and our grief. We can feel the intimate connection we have to all of life, and to the heavenly energy. When we stand in stillness and open to Shen, we feel the presence of a power greater than ourselves. Like the Tao, the Universal Loving Light is mysterious and beyond words.

From Stillness to Movement

Qigong and Tai Chi forms develop the capacity to maintain a constant, even flow of yin and yang energy. We move from empty to solid to empty. Our arms float up with the inhale and descend with the exhale. We sink into the solid grounding of the earth and receive the natural rising as an opposite reaction. Expansion returns to contraction and contraction becomes expansion. These waves of movement and vibration in our body drive out the kinks of muscle tension, calm our nerves and cleanse our organs.

The other day I was able to explore Sulphur Creek. It is a westward flowing stream which springs from the geysers in the Mayacamas Mountains and runs twenty miles to empty into the Russian River. I found a spot where I could go down to the water. The spring waters gushed and sparkled over the rocks and boulders making many small waterfalls and a powerful thundering sound. After some exploration I found a flat rock where I could sit comfortably below a stretch of waterfalls as they flowed into a deep pool.

We were three weeks into the Corona virus crisis with its stress and isolation. The news from New York where death had taken its worst toll was devasting. I couldn't forget the images of the struggling care workers and the mass graves. All I wanted was to just sit quietly and meditate.

Looking into the deep pool, my gaze continued across to the opposite bank where a thirty-foot, sheer, moss covered boulder rose out of the water. Its great form sat in stillness and became a reflection of returning stability within me.

I sat, watched, and listened to the rushing water. The sound pummeled my body and mind into softening. The sunlight warmed my skin in the coolness of the spring morning. I kept my seat for about an hour, just staying kindly with my emotions. At the end of my meditation, I washed my face in these natural flowing waters, giving myself a water blessing.

When I wandered downstream and up on the rocky bank, I found a fairly flat spot in sandy soil. Wanting to do

Qigong, I smoothed out a three-foot circle with a piece of driftwood and pounded the sand down with my feet. There were numerous golden colored rocks scattered throughout the riverbank. I picked up about thirty of them and placed them around the circumference. The golden rocks made my Qi circle glow.

Entering the circle center, I stood silently in Wuji. Breathing the crisp air, my whole body became one breath. I began shifting my weight with my breath, moving into Crane Flies, and several spontaneous Qigong movements. The routine ended with massaging circles, rubs, and taps. Putting my hands on my belly, feeling my whole-body tingling with Qi, I gave thanks to Mother Earth and Father Sky and my own life stream. The crisis was still there, but my heart and mind had expanded to embrace it with compassion and generosity.

FOUR

The Principles of
Intention and Virtue

Sifu Nam Singh expected his students to follow him without complaining. If you complained, he would work you so hard you would quit. The class started out with about thirty students and ended up with maybe a dozen. I never knew what to expect when I went to class. He was an unpredictable Water Dragon. No two classes were the same. Sometimes he would push our bodies to exhaustion. For example, he would make us do strenuous horse stances where we held a deep squat, our thigh bones parallel to the floor, for twenty minutes and more. Or, we would perform a series of 108 punches or other challenging fighting techniques. We had weapons practice using staves, sabers, and the classic double- edged sword. Occasionally he demonstrated intricate weapon forms and would fly around the room leaping, slicing, stabbing, and blocking.

Many times, Sifu would start class with twenty minutes of universal post or simple standing. We would hold perfectly still in cat stance, arms held out in front of our body making a big full circle of what he called Peng energy. After about ten minutes our arms would shake, and our legs would quiver. We felt we had to prove ourselves by maintaining the posture in perfect stillness.

My mind and body were saying I had to give up, I couldn't bear to hold the position anymore. I remembered Sifu saying, "Where the mind goes the Qi follows." I started directing my breath into my arms and legs. I felt a surge of spaciousness. My arms and legs became lighter and it was like the Qi was holding them up. I told my Sifu I felt myself cross a threshold in understanding about the power of Qi. "Good!" he said, "now you know it's not muscle strength, it's your intention."

Power of Yi

Yi is known as the power of intention. Martial artists say, Yi is the strongest power they use, not their fists, muscles, or weapons, but their intentions. Yi power focuses the Qi. When the mind focuses on a desired outcome, it can be like a laser beam of intense determination. Intention is a necessary component when martial artists are breaking bricks and boards with their fists. They think of their fist going *through* the brick, not *to* the brick. If their mind stops at the brick, they will likely break their hand, without breaking the brick.

I remember breaking boards with Sensei Gayle Fillman at Aikido class in her Ukiah Dojo. I was scared. I am a small person and a bit fragile with some arthritis in my precious hands and I hate getting hurt. But I lined up with the other brave novices and took my turn. I approached the pine board resting between center blocks. I took three deep breathes. With the first two exhales, I imagined my fist going to the other side of the pine board. On the third exhale, my intentional punch was released through the shattered board.

Yi force gives Qi direction and movement.

By our intention, our Yi, we move our Qi to reach our goal. Yi works with our imagination and our creativity. It is the energy we use for the manifestation of our desires. If a great idea comes to mind, from the depth of our desires and imagination, we can figure out how to put it into action through the power of our intention.

The Yi gives us the power to change our minds, our bodies, and our connection to spirit. The mind engenders our attitudes, but we can change our mind by changing our intention. Years ago, I suffered from depression and would lose myself in a dark swirl of fear, shame, and anger, sometimes for weeks. I wanted to get out of my depression. The last thing I wanted to do was go anywhere, but I knew Qigong class would help, so I showed up. Deep conscious breathing and moving my limbs and twisting my body in Qigong wrung out those stuck places. It was mysterious to me that I could move my body and change my mind. Qigong strengthened my body, calmed and cleared my mind. I found that I was suddenly happier.

If I wanted a better attitude to bring my energy up, another way I found helpful was making a gratitude list. A typical list might include the beauty of the blooming purple iris in my back yard, the well stacked wood pile, that my daughter was healthy and happy, that I had a Qigong class available. Instead of being immersed in my negative thinking, I shifted my attention to what made me happy, what worked for me.

"What we cultivate grows"

How we act and react to what comes our way is something we can develop over time. We have the power to change our behavior and not be a victim of our emotions.

Li was explained to me, by Sifu, as behavior. He said, a mother will say to her misbehaving child, 'Li, Li!' 'Watch your behavior!' Li is used as a command to bring attention to the child and what they are doing.

Li is also understood as the natural growth patterns of creation, from the grains and knots in wood and jade, to the evolutionary patterns found in DNA. Each living organism is unique and has its own natural unfolding. Li is the structure through which energy moves. It is the pattern energy uses to create form. Li is the "implicate order" we observe in the manifestations of Qi. We can become aware of our natural propensities and learn to guide our behavior to be more skillful.

We pay our respects to Li when we bow with the intention of "Kuan Li," as presented in Chapter Two. Kuan Li means "merciful behavior." It reminds us to respect to our own nature, to respect others' nature, and to honor the nature of heaven and earth.

Principles of Qi, Li, Yi and Te

There is no Qi without Li.
Li has no direction or life without Yi.
For culture to thrive, virtue, Te, is required.
The energy of Qi needs the order and the
structure of Li for manifestation.
For movement and direction, Qi uses intention, Yi.
Yet for success, Te is required.

Classic Chinese Qigong saying

Power of Te, the Essential Virtue

The great sage Lao Tzu said, "Not to part from
the invariable te, is to return to the state of infancy."
Te represents the inherent power of love and truth
within us, the purity of innocence.

Why I needed Tai Chi

I started my training in 1976, the Year of the Fire Dragon. My mother died of breast and bone cancer on January 7th that year. I was haunted by guilt for not fulfilling my mother's wishes. She wanted me to marry a nice doctor, have a nice house, and be a devoted good Christian. I was divorced. I had to work to support myself and my daughter. I was too poor to go back to school and get my degree. I distrusted marriage, I distrusted the system, and worst of all I distrusted myself.

I had broken the old standards of society and I was suffering from what my sister called, "death by a small town." So, I moved to Sonoma, California, and worked for four years at a state hospital for the developmentally disabled.

The doctors were all male. They were given what seemed to me an unfair amount of privilege and respect. They were paid three times what the nurses received, yet the nurses did most of the work. The nurses worked with the patients and knew what the patients required, but they would have to pander to the doctor to get the orders to do what was needed. Watching this, I became really angry with the subservient role of women in the workplace.

I quit working at the state hospital and started working with another woman as a potter. It was healing to work with clay, but the long hours also left me stiff and sore in my lower back and hands. In 1976 I started taking Tai Chi classes. In the midst of anger, exhaustion, and depression I would force myself to go to class. I would tell myself, "suit up and show up!" I started doing a daily practice, going to every class available, four days a week. I found that by moving my body in the Tai Chi way, I became more peaceful and contented. I learned the principle, "move your body, change your mind."

The Tai Chi principle of soft overcomes hard was the opposite of my previous exercise experience. Gradually, I learned to focus on relaxing without being floppy. Sifu said, "It's not about muscle strength, it's about energy." I learned softness wasn't weakness.

I was attracted to two principles. The first is Kuan Li, merciful behavior, acknowledged in the Tai Chi bow. The second is the basic Taoist principle of being in harmony with nature. I vowed to be in harmony with my own nature. I wanted peace in my troubled life. Was peace possible? What was my Li? Was my Li merciful?

The Women's Movement and Back to the Land

Along with a groundswell of other women, I joined the feminist movement in what was called the Second Wave of Feminism. Women were helping other women survive and escape the victimized roles we were given. This was chuan practice for me, taking responsibility for myself and refusing to be a victim. We started the Sonoma women's circle discussing needs and exploring solutions to common problems. We published a small paper. I joined Women in the Martial Arts and PAWMA. We were changing what it meant to be a woman.

In 1978, my partner and I, and my daughter Bridget, moved to the country. We bought a small cabin on 20 acres in Mendocino County, in the "back to the land" movement. We wanted to be self-sufficient and "in harmony with nature," exemplifying the Taoist motto. It was over two miles up an unpaved road with no power.

We brought goats. Goats provide the kind of milk that is more nutritious. People and other baby animals can drink it when they may be allergic to cow's milk. It is thought of as a universal donor like blood type O negative. Goat's milk is considered easier to digest. It enhances the body's ability to absorb important minerals, whereas cow's milk can block them. Goats are much smaller than cows and somewhat easier to manage. They are browsers and enjoyed the oak and madrone trees that were growing on our property. We also brought chickens for eggs, meat, and manure. We built a chicken coop and yard next to the garden so we could easily throw them greens and potato bugs, which they gobbled up with a flurry. A German friend brought us a pair of geese, which we named after her parents, Wolfgang and Marta. Marta became Bridget's pet and would follow her around which made us laugh. Our little farm was a dream come true. The organic garden flourished with the goat manure and alfalfa hay mix that Bridget regularly cleaned from the barn. About the only food we bought at the store was flour, honey, salt, and butter. That's about all we could afford. We were "dirt poor." Goat's milk makes wonderful cheese, but it is naturally homogenized and requires an expensive separator to make butter. For me, butter is a necessary luxury.

The shelter where the three of us lived was a shipping container, eight feet wide and forty feet long. It had been paneled inside and out, and remodeled with a door, windows and a small loft. That became Bridget's room. A fifty-gallon metal water tank rested on the roof. This was filled from a larger plastic tank that sat in the small creek at the bottom of the ravine. A sump pump powered by a gas generator drew water about 200 feet through a one-inch PVC line up the steep hillside to fill the roof tank. This fifty-gallon tank supplied the water for the livestock, the garden and personal use. One of us would have to go down to the creek to check that all the lines were intact before we started the arduous task of cranking the gas generator fast enough for ignition.

The garden soil was based on the compost from left-over food, pruning, grass cuttings, and good manure from the Nubian goats and the rabbits that my daughter raised in her 4-H program. We had milk and meat and lots of vegetables. I cooked on a cast iron wood stove that had two removeable plates on top. We didn't have electricity for about a year and used kerosene lamps and candles. In the cold, dark winter, we used a kerosene lantern to get to the goat barn, and to see to milk the goats. We had no phone, no TV, no radio, but we could hear the coyotes yipping down the canyon. We heard the wind, the birds, and the creek. In the evening we would talk, read, or play cards. Bridget and I would sometimes crochet or sew.

We got up before sunrise to do chores, have breakfast, and get my daughter off to school. She walked over two miles down the hill to the bus stop. Then I would go up the hill to a metal and wood building we'd built for a ceramic and graphic studio. Sue would work with the garden and animals most mornings before joining me in the studio. Our income came from ceramics we sold to art galleries and specialty shops, and Sue's illustrations commissioned for textbooks by McGraw Hill and other publishing companies.

The hardest part of life on the farm was losing an animal to sickness or injury. Our goat named Madrone died the first winter of pneumonia. The stress of the move combined with winter rain and cold were too much for her. It was devastating to hear her bellow in pain. The local vet came to our farm and put her down. We buried her crying. I wanted to quit. It was not the nice happy life I'd dreamed we'd have.

I was humbled. When we slaughtered an animal for meat, it reminded me that I depended on life for food that sustained us. We lived off life, whether it was a carrot or a chicken. I had a new appreciation for giving thanks in a prayer before I ate.

Permission to Teach

For a year I'd go back to Sonoma, about seventy miles away, to train with Sifu Nam Singh. I would get there for the evening class, spend the night at the temple and stay for the 7:00 AM morning class. Sifu would have me teach the warmups and help with the form corrections for his beginning students. As I shared information and skills with others, the teaching experience expanded my own knowledge. I noticed how Tai Chi, with its balanced harmony, strengthened the women and gentled the men.

In 1980 I began teaching on my own. Following traditional respect for a teacher, I asked Sifu if I could teach in my own community. He said, "Are you asking me or telling me?" I said, "Both." He said, "Well, OK then."

I started teaching my family and a few of my neighbors. I went across the valley once a week to teach the lesbian separatists on Green Wood Ridge at Lavender Hill. Eventually I taught in the largest town in Mendocino County, at Ukiah's Vinewood Park and the Redwood Health Club where I taught men and women.

In those days, women tended to retreat when men were present in class, and men tended to take over. As a feminist I wanted to empower women and held women-only classes for many years. When we women got together there was a special energy, a certain buzz of excitement, a mutual understanding and trust. When even one man joined the group, the energy changed. Women tended to make less of themselves so the men would shine. A sense of demureness shrouded the fullness of their being.

Many women gained confidence through their practice. The head of the local battered women's shelter said it helped her be patient in her stressful job. She has been able to hold her position there for forty years. Therapists began using the centering techniques for themselves and their clients. One woman said Tai Chi had helped her, in a custody battle to keep her children. She said every time she would do double-punch, she would think of her two kids, and her strong intention to keep them with her. She won the case.

Yi Projects Qi

The Power of intention is what gives Qi
purpose and direction.
Yi brings attention into focus.

> # "Where the mind goes,
> # the Qi follows"

Yi projects Qi. The basic Qigong principle is, "Where the mind goes, the Qi follows." Through our intention, we project and guide Qi in our own body for healing and can project Qi to heal others.

Through Yi we can send and receive Qi. The popular Japanese healing system known as Reiki utilizes projected Qi. The Reiki practitioner or master is a conduit for healing Qi.

Reiki is made up of two words. Rei is defined as: universal life energy, spiritual consciousness and all knowing. Rei is like the Chinese Yuan Qi or primal Qi energy. Ki in Japanese is like Qi in Chinese. It is breath, life force and vital radiant energy. The Japanese characters differ from the Chinese as the symbol is rain instead of steam. The rain falls on three open mouths representing prayer, breath and the expression of our truth. The lower ideogram of Rei is a king representing the ruler in each of us. Ki combined with Rei connects breath energy with spiritual consciousness and universal creative energy.

Reiki is hands-on healing with specific hand placements. Reiki Masters place their hands on or near the recipient allowing universal life energy to pass through their palms. Treatments can also be given to yourself or any life form. Like Qigong healing treatments, Reiki uses various sounds and symbols to induce healing. The masters connect with three levels of treatment corresponding to light, love and power. It is an energy treatment where two people connect in a meditative healing atmosphere. The subject may be in a lying or sitting position as they relax and open to the healing treatment.

It is understood that each person is responsible for his or her own healing. The healer is there to assist the process of restoration. It may be an emotional, physical, or a spiritual healing.

Both Reiki and Qigong project healing energy from the palms. Projected energy stimulates the area where the energy is received, inducing homeostasis and healing. The recipient actively receives the energy with the intention of creating wellness.

The idea of projecting Qi is illustrated by studies of Dr. Masaru Emoto, doctor of Alternative Medicine in Japan. He showed that a projected attitude and intent could change the molecular structure of water and snowflakes. Positive loving energy projections produced harmonious complete patterns and negative hateful energy projections produced broken deformed structures.

In China, a group of about six people did an experiment of projecting energy into two identical cylinders of cooked rice. In one they projected loving energy, and into the other hateful energy. The rice in the container that received positive energy was good, fresh and edible. The negative energy produced rotten inedible rice. We can use our thoughts to project loving Qi energy into our own body to restore health.

Traditional Chinese Medicine maintains that disharmony and blocks to Qi in the body result in disease. The treatment for disease is to increase free flowing energy in the meridians and to balance Qi in the body. The meridians of the body are thought of as rivers of Qi. Like water, when Qi flows, it's clean, clear and fresh. When the flow of Qi is stopped, it stagnates and creates decay and an environment for disease.

Practitioners use their mind, their hands or acupuncture needles to stimulate and restore the natural flow of Qi. Qi moves through the body, dissolving blocks and stagnation. Relaxation allows blood and lymph to flow more easily. Acupuncturists usually prescribe a good diet and herbs to support healing, often adding a Qigong practice specific to the patient's issue or illness.

The body is a servant to the mind. It will do the best it can to perform what we want until it wears itself out. In Qigong our mind is brought into the loving service of the body. By connecting to the loving light of Shen we integrate our mind, body, and spirit which creates the possibility for restoration and healing.

Qigong and Tai Chi treat the areas of disharmony and disease with stillness, meditation, gentle massaging and stretching techniques. We practice using Yi to restore wellness. We project our breath into the body to relax and heal. The mind guides Qi through the body. The flow of Qi releases tight joints and muscles and cleans and refreshes stagnant places, restoring health. When Qi flow is open, health is restored.

Trying Softer

Tai Chi practice helped me learn to try softer not harder. Sifu would have us stand in meditation stance, like the basic Universal Post stance, with our arms out as if we were embracing a tree. I learned after a couple of minutes that if I was stiff or rigid, I would get exhausted and have to give up my stance and let my arms down. However, if I relaxed and became soft, I had more stamina. If I kept my attention on my breath and breathed into my sore places, I would have the energy I needed to stand longer. I could feel my whole body breathing and filling with relaxed aliveness. The breath itself seemed to be holding me up and expanding into every part of my being.

The principle of "Try softer not harder," held true when I did the moving form of Tai Chi. If I was stiff, I'd lose my balance. Once I learned a specific movement and its application, I worked on being soft. Then I was grounded and more agile. In soft presence I was more alert to the energy and action around me. I notice the fluidity of my whole body coordinated with all the other people doing the form. Sometimes it felt like we became one animal moving in unison.

With my daily practice I became more aware of the subtle changes in the smell of the air, the sounds of machines, the songs of birds from day to day. Thoughts and sensations would come and go. Whatever was happening didn't really interfere with my continuous movements and breathing. Sometimes it was crisp, cold and clean or fragrant with lavender in bloom, the fresh pungent odor of pines or bay trees. Sometimes I could smell smoke from the neighbors' fireplace. I could hear the neighbors watering their garden and felt happy they have a garden.

Ultimately, I learned that by directing my mind into my body with intention, Yi Chuan, I changed the way I thought and moved. The neurons in the brain and throughout the body fire and move along the path of nerve bundles that are strengthened through use. We form habits by repetition. The more we repeat something the stronger it gets, whether it is physical, mental, or emotional. The simple daily practice of Qigong and Tai Chi made me calmer and more alert.

Te, the Highest Good

The concept of Te, virtue, is basic to Chinese philosophy. "What is the highest good?" is the question of Te. Lao Tzu says, "Not to part from the invariable Te is to return to the state of infancy." A fresh presence maintains the essential virtue of Te. Chinese philosophy believes Te is an inborn quality and the true original nature of humankind. The Chinese character for Te is a combination of the ideograms for a simplified foot combined with the modified characters for "true" and "heart." It is this true heart that upholds the Te.

When I was a child, I loved singing the lines of my favorite Lutheran hymn which read, "Create in me a pure heart, and renew a right spirit within me." We sang it with the opening liturgy in church every Sunday. It would bring me into the same place I now call Te.

We open our heart and can listen to its wisdom by relaxing and breathing into it. We direct and connect our mind with our heart to let the true Immortal Spirit, the Shen, guide us. The Shen is the Knower, The Deathless, the Loving Light. It is the part of our heart that is naturally compassionate. The Shen aligns with our conscience. Our conscience is both natural and learned. We are taught the difference between right and wrong according to our culture, but we also know it intuitively.

Being responsible for our actions and acting with integrity is the Chuan of Te.

Taking responsibility is the fist of Chuan.

Sometimes as I held the mudra, Chain Link of Grace, I would feel my right fist curled into my left hand. I remembered; the fist represents taking responsibility for myself. I could feel my fist of action covered by my left hand which represents my intuition, my inner teacher.

I started being more mindful about where I placed my attention. Was I nourishing myself and others or was I caught up entertaining blame and revenge? Or was I just entertaining to be liked? Was I being authentic? When I follow the path of the true heart by honestly listening to my heart–mind and body, I feel the presence and guidance of the loving light of Shen, and I find my Te.

Yi = intention, Li = behavior, Te = virtue

The Greatest Virtue is to be in Harmony with Nature

In our Western culture we are often taught that our nature is sinful and shameful. Nature is to be overcome, tamed, and conquered. In the West, virtue is usually acquired through heroic deeds and abstinence. Self-denial and renunciation of our original sinful self is seen as the path to virtue. In Eastern culture, Taoist philosophy teaches the highest good is to be in harmony with nature. Eastern tradition adheres to the idea that we are part of nature. Our Li is illustrated by the principle of living simply so that others may simply live. This gives us the possibility for correct relationship.

The interplay of our Jing and Shen energies creates our unique character. Our inherited Jing energy gives us our physical body. Shen is the spiritual energy that guides our heart and mind. The state of our Shen is revealed in our attitude and on our face as our expression. What we do with our Jing body and our Shen thinking develops our virtue or Te. When we are led by our Shen, we have virtue.

> **When we are led by our Shen, we have virtue.**

When I was young and going to the Lutheran church, I learned that the Holy Spirit is written in our mind and in our heart. I often felt the comfort and renewal of this spirit. But as an adult, I left the church because I was angry at the Christian church for its abuse of women, its judgements, and the shame it engendered. I had shut down to all spiritual belief systems and I felt sad and isolated. After several months of Tai Chi, I noticed changes in my attitude. The experience of Shen was so similar to the experience of the Holy Spirit, my anger towards the church softened. I felt more accepting of the flaws and appreciated the good the church offered.

I enjoyed moving my body. My self-consciousness diminished. I had fewer headaches and stomach aches. I stopped shaming myself. Moving in unison as a group in Tai Chi helped me be more forgiving of others. I felt more connected to life. I wasn't as afraid to talk to people or go on walks in the park by myself. My confidence in my ability to do things grew.

If human beings are to survive, connection to Shen is vital. If our Yi intentions are of greed and hate, we will only produce violence, pain and destruction. Without the loving light of consciousness and compassion, Te, virtue, and integrity are not attained. Virtue offers the rewards of a peaceful life, a life respectful of nature.

"Kuan Li" is Merciful Behavior
for all sentient beings.

Yi Chuan, I Chuan, Intentional Action

The power of intent is the strongest power in the martial arts. Yi Chuan, also spelled I Chuan, is translated as Mind Boxing or Intentional Fist. The Chuan fist of self-containment is not a fist of aggression. The practice of Yi Chuan focuses attention on a desired outcome and opens the way to get to that goal. I first learned of I Chuan at the woman's martial arts camp in the late 1970s from Sherry Jiang who led a workshop on it.

In June of 2016 I was asked to lead the closing session for the I Chuan Association in Sacramento by its president Dug Corpolongo who has a school in Albuquerque, New Mexico. I arrived at the I Chuan Conference in time for Dug's session of Yi Chuan. Dug was a very big man, a heavyweight champion and judge at push hands tournaments with many achievements and honors in the martial arts world. I bowed to Sifu Dug and went to the back of the room as they were already in session. I watched and followed his movements. They were subtle. He was standing in what I knew as Universal Post with slight adjustments of the arms and wrists. We held each stance about five minutes. He was using I Chuan standing method to increase expansive, internal force or peng energy. Peng energy is a yang energy. The arms are extended, forming a circle. The peng energy fills the area around the body and arms like filling up a big balloon.

After about half an hour of standing we took turns bouncing an opponent off our arms. Most of the participants were push hand students practicing the art of repelling an opponent with peng energy. One person would push against another person's arms held in posture of Yi Chuan and the pusher would be repelled away by the power of the expansive peng force. You could barely see the movement in the person projecting the peng energy. It was like the one doing the pushing received an electrical shock as they bounced away from the person who remained almost motionless in the Yi Chuan stance. Some practitioners were able to send the opponent several feet through the air without very much movement on their part.

That evening we went to the Asian Pearl Restaurant for a celebration of Grand Master Henry Look's 90th birthday feast. It was a grand affair with many of his old friends and students attending. The food was plentiful and exotic, including Peking duck, whole fish, and whole chicken with the head still attached. In Chinese tradition, it is considered good luck to serve the whole animal. There was an abundance of other traditional Chinese cuisine. I didn't always know what I was eating, but it was mostly delicious.

Before we were seated for dinner, people were gathering and looking at the two posters composed of many photos from the master's life. Henry Look had been a very successful architect as well as a Grandmaster of I Chuan. He was now retired and had suffered an illness that affected his speech and put him in a wheelchair. I noticed that no one was talking to him, so I went up to him to pay my respects. I bowed and told him who I was, and that it was an honor to meet him and to take part in the I Chuan Conference. I asked him about the photographs, which he was happy to talk about. He seemed to appreciate my attention and my respect for his achievements and delighted to tell of his adventures in China, and in Sacramento and San Francisco. I was very pleased that I was seated to his right side at dinner, and enchanted when he served me some of his beautiful fish.

Grand Master Look had quite a life. He was born in Sacramento in 1916 and moved to China with his family as a young boy. He said his parents wanted him to get a traditional Chinese education. He returned to the USA and worked in San Francisco as an architect. He studied martial arts, being trained by three Grand Masters. He excelled in Tai Chi Chuan, Hsing I, I Chuan, Bagua Chaung, Qigong and weapons, winning many awards. He said he advocated the five highest levels of achievement: Honor, Respect, Integrity, Loyalty, and Humility.

Master Look met with Madame Wang Yu-Fang while he was in China, and she asked him to establish the I Chuan Association in the USA. Madame Wang was the daughter of Grandmaster Wang Ziang-Zhai, who was responsible for formalizing the internal art called I Chuan. Henry agreed to bring the practice to America, and the I-Chuan Association USA was established in 2003, and now has members throughout the country.

The wonderful thing about I Chuan is that it is based on internal principles that advocate a strong yin. The practice is founded on a grounded, soft energy, which supports the peng energy. A strong yin produces a strong yang. Soft overcomes hard is the way of Tai Chi Chuan and I Chuan. These principles are exemplified in the standing practice of basic I Chuan, also known as Yiquan in pinyin.

> # A strong yin creates a strong yang. Out of stillness, comes movement.

Practice Seven:
I Chuan or Yi Quan

Each of the eight postures are held about five minutes.
This has been adapted from Grand
Master Look's handout.
I Chuan is a Wuji practice beginning with
connection to the Three Powers,
Heaven, Earth, and Breath.

Position 1: Place your feet shoulder width apart and
connected to earth. Your head is suspended and connected
to heaven. Your arms are in universal post position holding
an imaginary sphere in front of your body. Sense the
expansive peng energy filling up the space between your
arms. Your palms face in. Fingers are expanded apart. Your
palms are held below your chin line. Your wrists turn
slightly to angle your palms upward, enabling qi projection
from the Lao Gong point to the upper dan tien. Your
elbows are held at least two fists away from your body. Sink
your body weight downward to the lower Dan Tien. Your
spine is in alignment from the crown of your head to your
buttocks. Your knees are slightly bent toward the front of
your toes. Be comfortable without straining. This posture
is the same throughout the practice.

Position 2: From position one with your arms held at the
level just under the chin, turn your palms to project into
the middle dan tien, the Central Terrace of the heart.

Continue to imagine a sphere with peng energy, being held in your arms.

Position 3: Your arms drop to the midpoint between the chest and naval, the solar plexus. Continue to imagine a sphere with peng energy.

This area is considered the seat of the will power and intention. This is the level of the solar plexus, a dense cluster of nerves just below the diaphragm. The diaphragm separates the upper abdominal cavity from the lower abdominal cavity and the middle dan tien from the lower dan tien. When you inhale, the muscle of your diaphragm contracts or tightens and moves downward. This increases the space in your chest cavity, into which your lungs expand. When you exhale the diaphragm relaxes.

Position 4: Continue to imagine a sphere with peng energy. From position three, turn your palms to angle downward. Focus the Lao Gong point on the lower dan tien, the Sea of Qi.

Position 5: Continue to imagine a sphere with peng energy. Bring your arms up so the palms are in line with or higher than your nose and held out as if you were looking through binoculars.

Position 6: Continue to imagine a sphere with peng energy. Drop your arms to shoulder height and shoulder width apart. Your palms are held with the Lao Gong points facing each other.

Position 7: Continue to imagine a sphere with peng energy. Rotate your palms downward and move your arms down to slightly below your shoulder height, at the level of the heart, with your fingers pointing forward.

Position 8: Continue to imagine a sphere with peng energy. Drop your arms down to the lower dan tien with your fingers pointing slightly downward, making a V shape, towards earth, with your hands shoulder width apart.

These positions will cultivate internal strength and expansive energy. They may be practiced individually or in sequence.

FIVE

The Five Phases; The Elements

The Taoists were great scholars who categorized many things. In their effort to understand nature, they mapped and charted the seasons, the directions, the sun, moon, the planets, and stars. They studied colors, the senses, flavors, emotions, and the organs of the body. They tried to make sense of the world in which they lived: the body they inhabited, the unpredictable earth with its droughts and floods. From their mountain top observatories, they studied the mystery of heaven and its celestial bodies. Yearning to understand and share this great mystery of life, they started keeping track and writing down their findings. Their conclusions are based on Tai Chi: the play of opposites, yin and yang in vibration and harmony.

The findings of the ancient Taoists correlate with our own. Modern physicists have shown us that all matter is made of various patterns of vibration from atoms and molecules to planet and stars that are composed of bound energy. They are held in place by electromagnetic and nuclear forces which work on the principle of polarity, which is the basis of Taoist philosophy.

In Traditional Chinese Medicine matter itself is regulated by what is known as Wu Xing or the Five Elements. In the Yellow Emperor's Classic of Internal Medicine, it is stated that, "The Five Elemental Energies of Wood, Fire, Earth, Metal and Water encompass all the myriad phenomena of nature. It is a paradigm that applies equally to humans." The Five Elements combine in various ways in patterns of creation and destruction. The ancient Taoists created a symbol of a pentagram within a circle to represent these patterns.

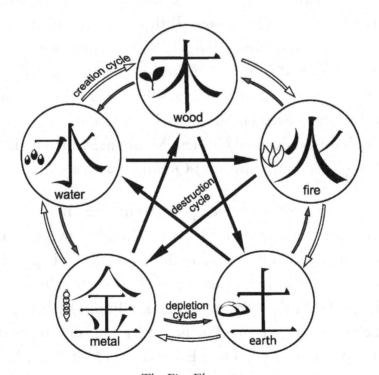

The Five Elements

The pentagram within a circle is the basic geometric pattern of evolving change in Chinese medicine. The five points of the pentagram star form a circle and represent the cycle of creation, and the pathways between the points that make the star represent the cycle of destruction. For example, in the creative cycle, symbolized by the circle, the element of fire creates the element of earth. In the destructive cycle, symbolized by the pentagram, the element of water destroys the element of fire.

Five Element Theory

The Five Element theory developed as a way to study and categorize basic manifestations, interactions and changes in nature. Qi energy creates all there is through the Five Elements or Wu Xing. The Five Elements, sometimes called the Five Phases, are cyclical in Traditional Chinese Medicine. They signify the ways in which Qi moves and acts. The study evolved into specific treatments and became the basis for Traditional Chinese Medicine, which includes herbology, acupuncture, and Qigong practice.

The cycle of creation, which goes around the circle, usually begins with the Wood Element. Wood represents the season of spring and new growth. Wood at the beginning indicates a recurring pattern as it is also the end of the cycle. In TCM they say, Wood makes Fire, Fire being the first element of creation. The next Element is Earth: as fire cools earth is formed. Then Earth makes Metal as it holds the Metal Element within it; metal ores are found deep within the earth. In this system Metal makes Water because water is carried by metal, as in metal pipes or vessels. And finally, Water makes Wood. As plants are watered, they grow. And again, Wood makes Fire, which begins another creation cycle.

In the destructive cycle, represented by the pentacle, Fire destroys Metal by melting it. Metal destroys Wood by chopping it. Wood destroys Earth by using up its nutrition. Earth destroys, or inhibits, Water by damming it. Water destroys Fire by putting it out.

The pentacle within a circle is not only an eastern symbol but a known symbol of other esoteric studies. It was revered by the witches of Europe, who were mostly Celtic clan healers, and used by the Kabalists in the Tarot. Like the dragon which is seen as a beneficial mythological animal in the east, the pentacle within a circle has been turned into something evil by some western Christians.

I have always been interested in religion and philosophy. Growing up Christian, I was also interested in Judaism, and the esoteric teachings of the Kabala. When I began studying Tai Chi and eastern ways of healing, I was surprised to find the same symbol of the pentacle enclosed in a circle. In Tarot cards, which evolved from the Kabalistic tradition, the symbol of the pentacle represents the suit of earth, which later became diamonds in our common card deck. Although there are many versions of the Tarot, I appreciate the classic Waite-Rider deck. It is based on Kabalistic symbols from the Bible and Torah and includes other concepts drawn from Celtic ideology, and the wisdom of the ancient Egyptians. I found the study of the archetypal symbolism in the Tarot fascinating. The various designs of Tarot integrated astrology, music theory, geomancy, and a host of other theosophical ideas. As the Tarot spread to other countries it acquired many variations, more of which are still being created.

The history of Tarot is uncertain. Some people believe during the Inquisition in Spain 500 years ago the persecuted Jewish Kabbalists and others disguised the then banned Hebrew Torah into a deck of cards and called it Tarot. The cards were based on the Hebrew alphabet and number system, so the Jews could study and worship and not be detected.

The Tarot has evolved over the centuries. The Major Arcana is comprised of twenty-two letters which are also represented by numbers. Some decks took out the Hebrew twenty-two letter-numbers of the Major Arcana, leaving only the Minor Arcana with its four suits. This is the standard card deck we have today.

The Waite-Rider Tarot deck is separated into the Major Arcana and the Minor Arcana. The Minor Arcana is separated into four elements: fire, earth, air, and water. These are the suits of the modern card deck with Clubs, Diamonds, Spades, and Hearts respectively. In the Tarot they are assigned to Wands, Pentacles, Swords, and Cups.

Noting similarities in distant cultures makes me wonder if this knowledge was shared by ancient travelers or just coincidence. It is reassuring to find that people from different places used the same symbols to describe their concept of the way things are.

Five Elements

"When the sage uses the five elements
in the right measure,
and in the most practical way, then they
can govern, or rule, or treat
without damage, loss or waste."
Huainaxzi 139 BC

The philosophy of the Five elements is based on the idea of Li as the model in heaven that reflects a pattern for mankind's behavior. Just as the celestial bodies move with regularity, and the earth has its seasons, so does humankind. The original Qi created form using the five elements. Each element has specific associations that connect to the Three Powers of Heaven, Earth, and Humanity. For example, Heavenly energy manifests as a sound, a color, or a season. Earth qualities are represented by functions of the body, our organs, and life cycles. Humanity is represented by our emotions, virtues, and mental preoccupations. These Five Element patterns describe a way to be conscious of our reality in form on earth.

Physiologically, each element is associated with a yin organ and a yang organ as well as a sense organ. Each organ of the body has a corresponding meridian. The yin organs are solid organs, and the yang organs are hollow. For example, in the Water Element, the bladder, which holds urine, is a hollow yang organ, and the kidneys, which filters blood, is more dense or solid and is a yin organ. The Fire Element's yang organ is the small intestines; it is paired with the heart, a solid yin organ. The yang organs tend to be containers where the yin organs are full of organic functions.

Five Element theory is the basis for many Qigong forms that stimulate the corresponding meridians and organs to harmonize their relationships to one another and bring the body into balance. According to TCM the five Elements are used to treat disharmonies in the body through diagnosis using the pulse and the appearance and condition of the patient. For example, if Wood is not producing Fire, the liver is not nourishing the heart, and this is shown by weakness, timidity, palpitations, poor memory, and insomnia. If the Fire is not producing Earth, the heart is unable to warm the spleen and there will be aversion to cold, cold limbs, distended abdomen, diarrhea, and edema. If the Earth is not producing Metal, the spleen is unable to nourish the lungs and there will be phlegm, and a cough. Metal not producing Water results in the lungs not sending water to the kidneys and there will be shortness of breath, thirst, weak knees, sore lower back. If Water doesn't produce Wood, the kidneys are not nourishing the liver and there will be tinnitus, low back pain, vertigo, tremors and emaciation. Diagnosis is also detected by the disharmonies that occur in the destructive cycle also known as the control cycle.

The Five Elements their Organs and Qigong

Wood

Even though the Wood Element is logically the last emanation of the cycle, the Five Element Theory generally begins with Wood because it represents new life. The Wood Element is associated with the season of spring which gets its life from the Water of winter. Its color is green, represented by the new green shoots. Its direction is East like the rising sun that starts the day. Wood represents new life energy that we feel in spring as we wake up from the cold dark winter. We fall in love in spring. We are spring fools, full of new plans and ideas.

In 1983 I took a partial live-in home care job for several years with a ninety-seven-year-old woman who had lived alone. She'd had a stroke that left her paralyzed in a wheelchair without the use of her hands or feet. She needed a lot of attention both day and night. I worked four days at a time each week. I was often exhausted. Sometimes I had trouble getting back to sleep after attending to her needs in the night. I was so sleepy during the day that it was difficult to function properly. I asked my Sifu what I could do. He said, "Put your mind in your liver." He explained: I was to direct my thoughts away from my anxiety about not getting enough sleep and think instead of my liver. He told me to visualize my liver as a big, dense, soft, floppy organ, and I would go back to sleep. I thought it was a strange treatment, but I found that it worked. At night, while we sleep, the liver cleanses the blood. By concentrating on the liver with our mind, we send Qi to the liver. Where the Qi goes the blood follows, so we can use our mind to direct energy into the liver and help the body put the blood where it belongs. The mind stops worrying as it is redirected into the breath and the liver and we naturally fall back to sleep.

Liver

The Wood Element is associated with the yin liver and the yang gall bladder. The liver is called "The General" because it is the master for the other organs and systems. It stores and filters our precious blood. It is associated with our vision. It governs the smooth flow of Qi. If the Qi is stagnant or blocked, we become emotionally frustrated and angry. We can feel stuck and powerless. The emotion assigned to the liver is anger. The antidote for anger is patience.

The soul, or hun, is thought to reside in the liver. According to TCM the hun is the part of our consciousness that contains our desires, plans, dreams, and imagination. At night, when we are sleeping, as the blood collects and is filtered by the liver, the hun gives us our dreams. In the day, our hun or soul looks out through our eyes. The eyes are the window to the soul. Taoists paid close attention to their dreams to increase their understanding of the messages from heaven. The soul and our shen are both parts of our consciousness.

Heart Mind Meridian Qigong

Heart Mind Meridian Qigong is a meridian form of Qigong which concentrates and directs Qi to flow throughout the invisible channels and organs of the body. I learned Heart Mind Meridian Qigong from its creator Matthew Swiegart at the National Qigong Association Conference in 2012. I was delighted because the meridians made sense for the first time. The forms include mantras that were created by Matthew for the various organs. He generously gave me his permission to teach the form with some modifications.

The mantra for the liver is,
"I envision my life with clarity and purpose."

Gall Bladder

The yang organ of the Wood Element is the gall bladder. The gall bladder is a muscular green sack located on the under-surface of the liver. It stores bile produced by the liver, squeezing it into the small intestine when food comes from the stomach and enters the duodenum. Its primary function is to break down fats. The gall bladder is one of the longest meridians, covering the body from head to toe. Both headaches and sciatica are related to the gall bladder. The Nei Jing states the characteristics of the gall bladder are like "an important and upright official who excels through his decisions and judgment." The gall bladder is influential in breaking down and ridding the body of toxins and promoting a more balanced state.

**The mantra for the gall bladder is,
"I stand my ground, with strength and integrity!"**

Fire

The spring ends and we move into the hot summer of the Fire Element. Its color is red. It can bring light, warmth, and happiness, or it can erupt, explode, burn, and destroy.

Heart

The yin organ associated with the Fire Element is the heart. The heart has the powerful energy of the Shen. Fire relates to our consciousness. It gives us our spiritual connection to Shen, which is called the Immortal Spirit or the Deathless. Fire gives us the energy we call love. Too much excitement or heart fire can manifest negatively in our emotions. The heart can feel so much stress that it can break. The antidote to negative fire energy is contentment. Qigong helps to quiet the heart fire and bring peace and contentment.

The Nei Jing Canon of the Yellow Emperor says, "The heart is the root of life and causes the versatility of the spiritual faculties. The heart influences the face and fills the pulse with blood." In TCM and Qigong the heart is known as the sovereign or monarch. The heart unites all the meridians so that their functions are coordinated.

Shen lives in heart and in mind. It's interesting that in the West we revere the brain and in the East the brain is rarely mentioned. In TCM the brain is not considered as one of the organs but a "Sea of Marrow." Shen acts as a filter for the greater consciousness of heaven which flows into our physical realm. Without filtering, the infinite information of the energetic realm would distract us or drive us insane.

Our personal consciousness connects to the universal consciousness through our heart-mind. When the mind is informed by heart Shen, we can experience the oneness of all.

Physiologically the heart is slightly larger than your fist and is well protected by the rib cage. It is a muscular pump consisting of four chambers. The right side receives the venous blood from the body by way of the superior vena cava and sends it to the lungs for oxygenation. The left side of the heart receives the oxygenated blood from the lungs and sends it into the aorta for circulation throughout the body. This loyal pump moves the blood through the body to provide nourishment to every cell, tissue, and organ. The heart pumps five or six quarts of blood each minute or about 2,000 gallons a day.

The Taoist view of blood is that it is the physical anchor and vehicle for Ying Qi and Shen. Ying Qi is translated as Nutritive Qi, the nourishing energy which travels with the blood and keeps the body functioning. Ying Qi movement corresponds to the flow of Qi through the organs during each two-hour period of the 24 hours of the day. It provides the Qi or oxygen from the air we breathe, and the nutrition needed from the food we ingest to nourish every cell and tissue of our body. Ying Qi nourishes because of its expansive quality which is a direct manifestation of the expansive nature of Fire element. The Fire Element travels with blood as blood is propelled by the heart.

In Tai Chi Chuan practice, after we connect to the Three Powers, we step out to our left, because the heart is on the left side of our body. We remember to move in the direction of our heart, to act with compassion, to have merciful behavior.

**The mantra for the heart is
"I am guided by my heart's inner truth."**

Small intestines

The yang organ of the Fire Element is the powerful small intestines. The small intestines break-up the food we eat into what the body can use and what it must eliminate. In TCM and according to the Nei Jing, the small intestines are like the "officials who are trusted with riches and create changes of the physical substance by sorting the pure from the impure." The sorting process is not only physical, but emotional and intellectual as well.

**The mantra for the small intestines is,
"I know what is false, and what is true,
and I keep what is true for me."**

Supplemental Fire

Pericardium

The Supplemental Fire Element is a helpful addition to the Fire Element. The yin meridian of this element is the pericardium, which is a membrane structure surrounding the heart that protects it. The Nei Jing says this is like "an official in charge of protecting the heart and guiding the pursuit of joy."

The mantra for the pericardium is, "I embrace the good way that nourishes my heart."

The Triple Warmer

Triple warmer is the yang meridian of Supplemental Fire. It is referred to as "the official in charge of regulation, of the temperature as it rises in the burners and strengthens the immune response."

The Triple Warmer has functional meaning for the organs but doesn't have an actual physical location. It controls Qi flow in the body as it ascends and descends, enters and exits. It controls the entire circulation of body fluid. The upper branches are located in the thoracic cavity and include the heart and lungs and respiration. The middle burner encompasses the spleen, liver, gall gladder, and stomach with the function of supporting digestion. The lower burner includes the kidneys, large intestine, small intestine, and bladder associated with the functions of supporting elimination.

Qi is transformed by the Triple Warmer. It is written in The Central Scripture Classic, Zhong Zang Jing, "The Triple Burner stems from the Yuan Qi (Primal Qi). It governs all Qi in the body. It has a name but no form." (Nan Jing Chapter 38.)

The Triple Warmer governs the flow of Qi, Shen and Jing. It takes Primal Qi and separates it into its different functions. It controls the movement and passage of Qi through Ying Qi or nutritive Qi, Wei Qi or protective Qi, and the blood and bodily fluids. Zong Qi (Gathering Qi) is in the upper Warmer. Ying Qi (Nutritive Qi) originates from the Middle Warmer. Wei Qi (Protective Qi) originates from the Lower Warmer.

When the Qi of the Triple Warmer has free passage, Qi moves easily in the body, into interior, exterior, left, right, above, and below. It irrigates the body and harmonizes movement of Qi.

**The mantra for the triple warmer is,
"I protect this precious life that I've
been given from all harm."**

Earth

The Earth holds the power of gravity. Our connection to earth establishes our center and our axis. It is the point of reference for our balance. When we align with earth energy in balance, we are free of stress because we have the ability to relax. Stress causes disease. In TCM it is understood that if earth energy is balanced, homeostasis will be maintained, and our body will be healthy.

The Earth Element connects the other elements, just as all life is connected to the earth. The Earth Element nurtures, supports, and interacts with each of the other elements. All living things emanate from and return to the earth. Therefore, the earth occupies the center and is thought of as abundant and beautiful in its natural harmony. Yellow is the color for the Earth Element. It was the divine color of the emperor as the Son of Heaven or Tian Zi. No one else could wear the royal yellow. The emperor's duty was to be "Heaven's Mandate" on earth. This was important because he moderated between heaven and earth.

Positively, earth energy denotes harmony, fairness, and instinct. Its negative quality is worry and has a smothering effect.

Spleen

The spleen is the yin organ of the Earth Element. It is located in the upper left abdominal region protected by the lower part of the rib cage. It is soft and about five to six inches long and two or three inches wide. The spleen contains lymph tissue for filtering worn out blood cells from the blood. Along with bone marrow, it produces white blood cells, antibodies, and stores blood for use in emergencies. The spleen is stimulated by impulses from the sympathetic nervous system and by epinephrine from the adrenal glands. The spleen is strongly activated in emotional states and in times of physical stress. The spleen meridian governs the pancreas which produces insulin and other enzymes that aid in digestion and maintaining our blood sugar levels.

Chinese tradition says that the spleen is partially responsible for moving and transforming food and distributing the energy from food. The spleen meridian travels through the stomach and up into the lungs to unify the Qi of food and air. It is therefore an important meridian for the production of a person's vital energy. The spleen unifies the blood.

The spleen mantra is,
"I love sweetness and I nourish
myself and others."

Stomach

The stomach is the yang organ of the Earth Element. It is a hollow organ just below the diaphragm. It stores the food we eat, helps with digestion, and purifies whatever we ingest with its digestive secretions. TCM considers the stomach the Sea of Nourishment. The meridian passes close to the sense organs and is affected by stress. It serves as a detector for emotional distress.

**The stomach mantra is,
"I know what I want, and what I
need, and I know how to get it."**

Metal

In the west we don't use the Metal Element; however, the Five Element theory was created in the Bronze Age when improvements in metal working made more sophisticated weapons. They also made great vessels used in the worship of the ancestors, often with inscriptions of events, people, or territory.

In contrast to the expansiveness of Fire, Metal is contracting and cold in nature. Its color is white. The Metal Element is complementary to the Air Element of the West. We can see the similarity in the suit of Swords in the Tarot. The air signs are associated with communication and are depicted in the Tarot as Sword. Metal represents the mental aspect, our intellect and our rational thought. Correspondingly, in TCM the Metal yin organ is the lungs, the organ of our breath. Breath is translated as Qi. It connects us to Heaven and Earth. If breathing is efficient, the Qi will be led smoothly through the body by the mind.

Fall is the season of the Metal Element. It is a time of gathering in, stocking up, and a time of leaves falling, a time of decay and composting, letting the old pass away.

The emotion associated with Metal is grief and sadness. Grief is actually an expression of love. The antidote to grief is courage. We suffer the loss of a loved one or an ability we can no longer perform because of an illness, injury, or aging. It takes courage to feel love, to let go of attachment, and come back into balance. Addiction and self-destructive behavioral patterns are associated with Metal. We cover our grief with substance abuse, which leads to more depression.

Lungs

The yin form of Metal is the lungs. According to TCM the lung meridian is activated in the early morning from 3:00 to 5:00 AM. This is the traditional time for meditation. Lungs bring in oxygen, a substance our body needs for the health of every cell. With each exhale, the lungs help to expel pathogens from our body.

Our skin is connected to this respiratory process. Our skin also breathes by absorbing heat and expelling sweat. This regulates our body's temperature. The skin is the biggest organ of the body. It is a protective shield from disease and physical harm, and it's equipped with sensory nerves. Its ability to feel physical sensation, and connection to the nervous system, links it to the Metal Element.

**The mantra for the lungs is,
"I breathe in the pure Qi from the
universe into every cell of my body."**

Large Intestine

The large intestine is the yang organ of the Metal Element. The large intestine helps to transport, transform, and eliminate surplus solid matter of what we ingest. It is known as the "Drainer of the Dredges." The muscular walls of the large intestine, which includes the colon, push the solid waste along and absorb water and nutrients. If the large intestine is not functioning properly, toxic wastes accumulate throughout the body and every system can be affected.

Constipation or diarrhea may be experienced on a physical or on a mental level. Energetically, the large intestine's role is to let go physically, mentally, and emotionally. If we hold on to a relationship that is harmful, if we hoard things or if we can't let go of old painful situations, the large intestines can be affected. Indigestion may cause confusion or depression in our mental state. Headaches and dental problems can also be a symptom of digestive problems. Health of the large intestine depends on how well we can let go of the difficulties in our life and move on.

**The mantra for the large intestine is,
"I gratefully let go of that which
I no longer need."**

Water

The Martial Arts Master, Bruce Lee, said, "To be a great fighter, be like water."

Water is yielding, but all conquering. Water extinguishes fire. Water wears away rock and corrodes metal into dust. It yields to overcome. It is the cradle of life. It seeks the lowest places and overcomes all.

The color for Water is black. Its season is winter. The negative emotion associated with Water is fear. The antidote for fear is clarity. When water rages in storms of destruction, it brings chaos and fear; yet when clear and calm, it becomes a reflective pool for our deep meditations. Clarity brings understanding; understanding brings compassion. When we have clarity, we can release our fears and take positive action.

Our fears are the flags to find the action we need for resolution. In Qigong and Tai Chi, we learn to embrace our fears. This is reflected in the Tai Chi movement Embrace the Tiger. As we bring the energy into our heart center, we bow. We embrace the places that scare us to find healing for our pain.

Our deep unconscious mind stores the memories of time and the stories our mind makes up. The subconscious holds our pain in wait for healing. If we don't take care of the snares and tangles and false stories of the subconscious, the stress on our body will cause illness. Cleansing the body of stress and blocks, and getting rid of old toxic energy, is largely the job of the waters of the body. We are mostly water. Qigong medicine flushes the toxins out of the body and mind by cleansing movements, massaging specific energy areas, and relaxing and projecting healing Qi with our mind.

Water is Yin.
Water is associated with the feminine all over the world.
Mother Earth is mostly water.
She is the dark goddess,
The Goddess of the depths, the subconscious, the hidden.
She is receptive to the Will of Heaven,
the Implicate Order of the Tao.

Kidneys

The kidneys are the yin organ of the Water Element. They store the Jing, the inherited energy of our ancestors in the Gate of Life (Ming Men.) Jing is the substance that provides organic life. It contains the possibility of birth, maturation, decay, and death. Kidneys are considered the root of life. The kidneys are the mansion of fire and water, the residents of yin and yang, the channel of death and life. They are a vital organ as the great filter for the waters of the body. Kidney failure is a step closer to death, because the body cannot survive if it has more toxins that it can get rid of.

In TCM tradition yin and yang, in the form of water and fire, are used to balance and harmonize the body. Water Element energy resides in the kidneys like lakes. The Gate of Life (Ming Men) includes Ming Fire which warms the water into steam. The steam rises up the length of the spine through the thrusting channel. At the top of the head, the steam turns into rain and pours down through the body to provide nourishment to the lungs before descending back to the kidneys.

The kidney meridian begins at the bottom of the foot, at the Bubbling Spring or Yong Guan. It is the point of sending and receiving energy to and from the earth. It flows up the inside of the legs, through the genitals, (where we get our ancestral Qi), into the kidneys themselves, and up to the Toxic Release point below the clavicle in the little hollows next to the sternum.

The kidney mantra is,
"I feel the vital life force energy
flowing deep within me."

Bladder

The bladder is the yang organ of the Water Element. The bladder meridian is one of the longest meridians in the body, starting at the eyebrow and going over the top of the head, down both sides of the back, down the outside of the legs, to the little toes.

The mantra for the bladder meridian is,
"I am driven to achieve, and I
keep an eye on my back."

Walk Through Time

We've come a long way from the sea's creation of DNA,
From the beginning of life on this planet.
A long time for earth to cool from the fires of creation,

Leaving metals to advance our civilization.
It took time for water to settle and clear,
For land to receive the seeds,
For trees to grow in the forest primeval,
For the garden of earth to prepare for our birth.
Only a few thousand years ago we
started waking up and asking.

Meridian Flow

The channels and meridians of the body are energetic pathways, like invisible rivers of Qi, flowing between and through the acupuncture points, source points, gates, and organs of the body. The points are where we can access the channels and meridians. Both acupuncturists and Qigong practices stimulate the meridians. They do this through acupuncture needles, massage, or by focusing the mind.

Meridian energy moves like a snake through the body. The points are found in little hollows that you can massage and stimulate. Rubbing the points and doing deep breathing opens the flow of Qi and brings harmony and health.

Each of the organ meridians support the flow of Qi to an organ and its energy points on a daily cycle of connection. The daily schedule starts at 3:00 AM to 5:00 AM with the lung meridian. This is auspicious, known as the hour of "Sweet Dew". Quiet and dark, this is the best time for meditation. The Heavenly Dew is forming on the receptive earth.

Sifu Nam Singh told me that the Bottle of Sweet Dew is often depicted in statues and paintings of Kuan Yin, the Goddess of Fearless Compassion. The potion she holds in her hands is offered for healing all ills. This power is given to us when we meditate sitting in calmness, breathing, and chanting. We accumulate the Sweet Dew of Heaven through the practice of meditation. Connecting to the time of the healing dew is powerful medicine. It is the time of breath, lungs, and the Element of Metal. The lung points 1 and 2 are located by the shoulders under the clavicle bone, one above the other.

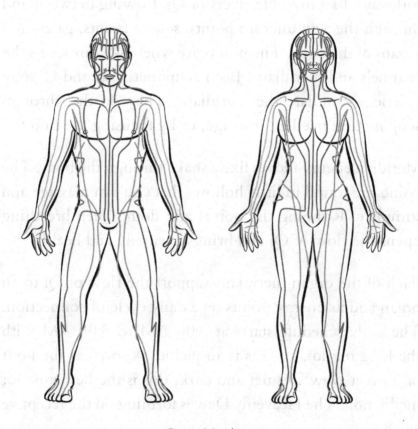

Organ Meridians

The Meridian Qi continues its flow from yin Metal and the lung meridian, to yang Metal and the large intestine meridian. The lung meridian flows from lung 1 and 2, down the inside of the arm to the thumb. This meridian is activated until about 5:00 AM and then the energy jumps to the index finger, the large intestine point and moves up the outside of the arm, up the neck, and ending at the outside of the nostrils. This large intestine meridian is especially active between 5:00 AM and 7:00 AM. This is a good time to have a bowel movement.

The energy then moves to the Earth Element and yang stomach. It starts just under the eyes and down to the second toe. It is active between 7:00 AM and 9:00 AM. This is when we start looking for something to have for breakfast. From 9 Am to 11 AM the energy moves to yin Earth and the Spleen, flowing from the side of the big toe and up into the Embrace Point in the lower ribs. It is usually an active, productive time. This is followed by the Fire Element, the yin heart, which starts in the arm pit and goes down the inside of the arm to the inside of the little finger. At noon we are at the center of heart energy, a time when there are no shadows, a time of truth.

Yang Fire from 1 PM to 3 PM is the time of the small intestine, which starts at the outside of the little finger and goes outside the arm, up the neck and to the face in front of the ear. At 3 PM meridian Qi moves to the beginning of the eyebrows for the bladder meridian that goes up over the head and all the way down to the little toes for yang Water. Yin Water and the kidney meridian, 5 PM to 7 PM, starts under the feet at the Bubbling Spring. It moves up the inside of the legs, through the genitals, the Ming Men, and to under the clavicle. From 7 PM to 9 PM the energy moves into Supplement Fire and the yin pericardium meridian, moving from the chest down the inside of the arm to the middle finger. It moves to the ring finger and up the outside of the arm to the outside of the eyebrow for the illusive, non-organ Triple Warmer from 9 PM to 11 PM. The energy at midnight from 11 PM to 1 AM is yang Wood and the gall bladder, which starts at the corner of the eye and zigzags to back of the ear, up to the forehead down the shoulders. It switchbacks down the ribs and the legs to the fourth toe. The cycle is complete in the dead of night with yin Wood and the liver meridian from 1 AM to 3 AM, a time of dreams. The meridian Qi moves from inside the big toe, up the inside of the leg and the groin, to the ribs below the nipple.

12 Meridians Qigong

from Matthew Sweigart HeartMind Meridian Qi Gong NQA 2012

Lung, Yin, Metal, 3-5 am (clavicle chest point 1, inside arm, to thumb 11)

I breathe in the pure Qi of the universe, to every cell of my being.

Large Intestine, Yang, Metal 5-7 am (index finger 1, outside arm, to outside nose 20)

I gracefully let go of that which I no longer need.

Stomach, Yang, Earth 7-9 am (under eye 1, down cheek, neck, nipple 17, close to body center across groin to over femur to 2nd toe 45)

I know what I want, and what I need, and I know how to get it.

Spleen, Yin, Earth 9-11 am (big toe 1 inside leg up to groin 12, outside nipple line to embrace 21)

I love sweetness, and I nourish myself and others.

Heart, Yin, Absolute Fire, 11-1 pm (arm pit 1, inside arm to little finger 9)

I am guided by my heart's inner truth.

Small Intestine, Yang, Absolute Fire 1-3 pm (little finger 1, outside arm to cheek and outside ear 14)

I know what is false and what is true, and I keep what is true for me.

Bladder, Yang, Water, 3-5 pm (eye inside brow 1, over top head, down center back, sacrum, back of leg to small toe 67)

I am driven to achieve and I keep an eye on my back.

Kidney, Yin, Water 5-7 pm (bottom of foot 1, behind knee 10, up center through genitals to clavicle 27)

I feel the vital life force energy flowing deep within me.

Pericardium, Yin, Supplemental Fire 7-9 pm (chest 1 down inside arm to 9 middle finger)

I embrace the good way that nourishes my heart.

Triple Heater, Yang, Supplemental Fire 9-11 pm (ring finger 1 outside arm to 23 end of eye brow)

I protect this precious life that is given to me from all harm.

Gall Bladder, Yang, Wood, 11-1 am (eye corner temple, back of ear, back up to forehead, then across the top of head to shoulder 21, switchbacks ribs in front, and then back to dimple in buttocks then outside leg to the fourth toe at 44)

I stand my ground with strength and integrity.

Liver, Yin, Wood, 1-3 am (Inside big toenail 1, inside leg groin 11, 12, bottom rib 13, below nipple 14)

I envision my life with clarity and purpose.

Five Animal Frolics

My Tai Chi sister Michelle Dwyer would say, "Nam Singh's class is always interesting. You never know what rabbit he'll pull out of his hat!" It seemed he had some new and interesting treasure to share every week. One of my favorite practices was the Animal Frolics.

The Animal Frolics are attributed to a famous acupuncturist and surgeon, Hua Tua, who lived about 2000 years ago in the Han Dynasty. It was a time of the Golden Age of Chinese medicine. In his study of nature and illness, he realized that disease could be prevented through diet and exercise. He noticed that animals that lived in harmony with nature were rarely sick. He designed exercises to mimic the movements and strengths of five animals which coincide with the five vital organs of the body and stimulate the specific organ's meridians.

I have seen and practiced many versions of the Animal Frolics with various teachers. The one I include here is moderate in complexity, and good for stimulating the organ meridians.

Sounds vary greatly among traditions. The important aspect is to breathe out and make a sound. This sound creates a vibration. The vibration can be directed into the meridian and organ for cleansing and strengthening. You want to feel the sound. The volume isn't important; it's the vibration that stimulates.

Practice Eight: Five Animal Frolics

Tiger: Element – Metal Organ – Lungs Emotion – Grief/ Courage

Movement: Stand with your feet shoulder width apart. Lean over and relax the lung meridian, letting your arms dangle. Make your hands into Tiger claws to stimulate the lung meridian, thumb to shoulder. The claws pull up energy from earth with the inhale as you rise; claws turn into soft fists at chest level. Return to claws as you exhale reaching up. Pull down energy from heaven as you return to soft fists at your chest level while you inhale. Breathe deeply and work the lungs. The exhale produces a soft "hhhaaa" sound vibration.

Bear: Element – Water Organ – Kidneys Emotion – Fear/ Clarity

Movement: Stand with your feet shoulder width apart, knees bent. Feel the Bubbling Spring at the bottom of your feet. In this movement the fists circle the whole abdomen as the body leans over and bends back, working the kidneys. It opens the kidneys as you lean forward and squeezes them as you lean back. Soft fists touch each other at the upper abdomen. The fists follow the motion of the body. Turn your upper body left. Bend forward and the fists slide down the left side of the belly with the exhale. As your waist turns to the right, the fists move across the lower abdomen. The inhale begins as you rise up. The fists move up the right side. As the fists move across the upper belly the upper body bends back. Complete the movement as you come to the top of the circle. Repeat two or more times then reverse direction. Inhale up and exhale down. Exhale has a soft "hhhun" sound vibration.

Deer: Element – Wood Organ – Liver Emotion – Anger/ Patience

Movement: Stand with your feet shoulder width apart with your arms relaxed at your sides. This movement is a twist and stretch of the body that stimulates the liver. Make antlers by bringing your third and fourth fingers into your palm. The thumb, index, and little finger stick out. The arms keep about the same distance apart. As you shift your weight left, your arms sway up to the left. The arms stretch out, the left arm is above your head, and the right arm is about shoulder height. Feel the stretch in you ribs. Sway to the right, shifting your weight as your arms come up at right side. Your left foot steps out into a lunge, stretching the liver meridian up the inner leg. Most of your weight is on your left foot. Continue to twist left, bringing your outstretched arms to your left side. Your right arm is overhead, stretching the right side. Your left side is compressed or closed. Look behind you, the antlers and fingers point in the direction of your gaze. This opens your right waist and closes your left waist, working the liver. Bring your weight back to the right foot, moving your arms back to your right side. Step back to the starting position with your left foot. Repeat on the right side. The exhale sound vibration is "ssshhh," quiet like a deer.

Monkey: Element – Fire Organ- Heart Emotion – Excitement/Contentment

Movement: Stand with your feet closer than shoulder width, crouch down, your arms dangling in front of your body. Open your arm pits and the heart meridian. Imagine your hands grasping peaches, palms down (Monkey steals the Immortal Peach). This stimulates your heart meridian. Inhale and rise up turning your hands into Eagle's Beaks (fingers together, pointing down) at heart level. Standing on your toes by raising your heels up. Your elbows are in by your ribs. Exhale and tilt your head to the left as your eyes look up to the right and then tilt your head to the right as your eyes look left. Return to center and lower your heels. Exhale sound is soft "hheyy."

Crane: Element – Earth Organ – Spleen Emotion – Worry/ Harmony

Movement: Stand with your feet more than shoulder width apart and your arms down at your sides. Feel the inner side of your foot and the outside of your big toe. Inhale and bring the left foot into a cat stance. Elbows down, wrists up, like big bird wings your arms rise to shoulder level at your sides. Exhale and drop your hands down in front of your body. Inhale as your wrists lead up again at your sides. As your left knee rises level with your hips it stimulates the spleen meridian. Exhale as you drop your wrists and bring your foot back to cat stance. Inhale and lift your arms over your head, with the back of your hands together, as your left knee comes up, Crane Spreads its Wings. Exhale keeping the weight on your right foot, your left foot returning to the original stance, reaches out to more than shoulder width. Settle your body down, weight still on the right foot; and then, shift your weight over to your left foot. Repeat on the other side. Exhale sound vibration is a soft "eeehhh."

Closing: Sink the Qi. Stand with your feet shoulder width apart. Your palms are open and facing down to feel earth energy. Your body sinks down slightly with a complete exhale. Soon you will feel your body wanting to rise up and fill with Qi. With the inhale the arms rise, led by the wrists. Your arms are held out to your sides at heart level. As you hold your breath, rotate your wrists and bring hands in gathering Qi to make a Qi ball. Receiving Qi bring the ball towards your solar plexus. With the exhale, rotate your wrists, and push your hands down sinking the Qi through the lower dan tien, (Sea of Qi,) and into the earth.

Sinking the Qi
centers and integrates the meridian
work of the Animal Frolics.

The Five Element Chart

Category	Wood	Fire	Earth	Metal	Water
Color	green	red	yellow	white	black
Flavor	sour	bitter	sweet	pungent	salty
Climate	windy	hot	damp	dry	cold
Development	sprouting	blooming	ripening	withering	dormancy
Direction	East	South	Center	West	North
Season	Spring	Summer	Late Summer	Autumn	Winter
Yin Organ	liver	heart	spleen	lung	kidney
Yang Organ	gall bladder	sm. int.	stomach	lg. int.	bladder
Sense Organ	eye	tongue	lips	nose	ears
Secretion	tears	sweat	saliva	mucus	urine, sexual fluids
Emotion	anger	joy	worry	grief	fear
Positive	patience	contentment	harmony	courage	clarity
Animal	deer	monkey	crane	tiger	bear
Sounds	sshhh	hheyy	eehh	hhhaa	hhhun

SIX

Dance of Harmony

Heaven above us
Earth below
We stand as members of Humanity

Breathing with all life
Integrating our mind body and spirit
As above so below

Everything is connected
We swim in the ocean of Qi
All changing in harmony

Moving between Heaven and Earth
We practice graceful continuity
Slowly with balance, clarity, and calm serenity

We dance with Qi
Breathing to the rhythm of the universe
Keeping time with eternity

Prelude to the Dance

Staying

It was the beginning Tai Chi class in the upstairs room of the old Sonoma middle school building. When I quietly closed the heavy wooden schoolroom door, slipping in to take a place in the back row, people were already standing in silence. Sifu Nam Singh was standing in front of the room.

He was a young, tall black man, elegant in his white raw silk Chinese jacket and black pants. His arms extended in front of his chest, with his beautiful long hands gracefully held, palms facing his heart. His eyes were softly looking through the small space between his fingers. He stood upright yet relaxed, in a pose with most of his weight on his back foot, and the ball of his front foot on the floor with his heel slightly raised in its black Chinese slipper. His head was crowned with a black satin cap supporting a red tassel. Facing him were over a dozen students who reflected his cat stance, their arms poised in the Hug a Tree or Universal Post posture. I took the position.

After a few minutes standing with knees bent, my thighs engaged and my shoulders began to relax as I breathed into my heavy arms stretched out in a circle before me. The stillness within the room and within myself created an internal action. My mind's focus moved naturally into my breath; it was all that was moving. I looked into my palms and studied my hands, continuing to listen to my breath. I felt a tightness, a pain in my shoulder. My thigh muscles were tiring from the unfamiliar low stance, knees bent just over the toes but not beyond. I was uncomfortable. Searching for relief, I breathed into the affliction, into my shoulder. I sent loving attention to open the space. My body started to relax.

I wondered what I'd cook for dinner, if I left the light on at home, and if I put the cat out. I became curious about the other people in the room. What did they do for a living? Were they married? How old were they? After about ten minutes, I wondered how long we were going to have to keep this up.

I realized that my mind was wandering. I brought my mind back into my body, to be with the stillness. I concentrated on my breathing, training my mind to come back into my body, into my breath.

Tightness and stiffness became the enemy to staying and keeping my position. I had to relax to survive. Fighting the discomfort, I wanted to give up. Giving in to the pain meant quitting. Holding and staying in posture required relaxation.

Holding and Staying require Relaxation

"SOFT OVERCOMES HARD," I could hear the Tai Chi principle in my mind. I had to breathe into the pain for relief. My breath allowed my body to come into unity, with all its parts, and stabilize me. Holding and staying was building strength in my arms and legs. I could feel my muscles shake. The man in shorts in front of me was also quivering. It was a struggle. My mind was telling, me just give up, let go, you can't do this, it's too much. But when I directed my breath into my limbs, it gave me strength to stay.

The breath itself was holding me up. Most of us held our ground. A few people dropped their arms and straightened their legs for relief. The standing practice lasted about twenty minutes. Sifu did a closing by relaxing his hands down to his belly. We did the same and we all relaxed. We all took a few big satisfying breaths. A flood of relief and elation washed over me. I felt like I had just passed a big test.

Learning to stay in posture, anchoring the mind and body with the breath, is an essential skill in Qigong and Tai Chi.

What's the difference between Qigong and Tai Chi?

Qigong and Tai Chi are based on the same principles of working with yin/yang to heal and harmonize the body-mind-spirit through specific forms that move the Qi. Qigong forms range from standing and stillness to short, choreographed movements that are often repeated several times. There are movements designed for specific conditions like relieving shoulder pain, helping digestion or activating the meridians.

Tai Chi Chuan is a much longer series of choreographed movements based on basic postures and their interpretation by the different schools, families, or masters that practice them. These postures include Single Whip, Wave Hands Like Clouds, Working the Shuttle, Grasping the Sparrow's Tail, Crane Stands on One Leg, Repulse the Monkey, Phoenix Spreads its Wings, and Snake Creeps Down. Even though their execution can vary greatly depending on the lineage and the master they are recognizable in any form.

The Classics: Organ Washing, Tendon Changing

Qigong is rooted in prehistoric times. The shamans and tribal leaders would communicate with the Three Powers of Heaven, Earth, and Humanity, leading the people in the Great Dance, Da Wu. Da Wu was done to heal, restore and strengthen the people.

Every Tai Chi class I've ever attended begins with Qigong practice, even if it's only knee circles. The only time Tai Chi is done on its own would be for a performance or demonstration and then it's done at "demonstration speed," which means a little faster than usual. Qigong is the warm up for Tai Chi. Qigong prepares the body, mind, and spirit to have a deeper, more relaxed, and present Tai Chi practice. Qigong invigorates the blood, warms up the muscles, tendons, and joints. For a smoother Tai Chi experience, Wuji Standing centers the body, mind, and spirit.

Qigong generally starts with Wuji practice of Simple Standing to connect with the Three Powers of Heaven, Earth, and Humanity. For moving energy and breath Wuji can expand into any number of practices. Qigong moves the energy throughout our meridian system. It massages the organs and glands in the classic practices of "Organ Washing" and strengthens the joints and sinews with "Tendon Changing" moves. Qigong uses stretching the muscles and massage to stimulate all systems, especially the circulation of blood and lymph which supports the immune system. Qigong practice often works with the meridian system. It is prescribed by doctors as a treatment for various illnesses or conditions.

Hui Tuo

Qigong is well documented with specific forms from about 2000 years ago. Hui Tuo, a great physician, is credited with creating several forms that are popular today including the classic Animal Frolics and Ba Duan Jing or Eight Brocades. One classic stance is called Shoot a Hawk. It takes a horse stance, which is a wide stance with rounded legs, as if one were on a fat horse. Just like a Mongolian archer, the arms mimic drawing a bow to shoot an arrow off to the side. Qigong often has a martial aspect. Many of the movements were created to keep the troops strong and healthy for the armies of the emperor. I have seen several different varieties of the Eight Brocades with similar movements, noting the changes that get made over the centuries as interpretations vary with generations of teachers.

Chang San Feng, Tai Chi Founder

Chang San Feng is considered the founder of the great dance of Tai Chi. He was a Taoist monk, scholar, and warrior in the time of the Mongol invasion of China in the thirteenth century. He sought to be in harmony with nature through a series of movements performed slowly and in a continuous flow. Making it a dance of philosophy, Chang set the forms to coordinate with the Eight Directions and trigrams of the Ba Gua, the foundation of the I Ching. Many movements in Tai Chi depict animals, reflecting the Taoist's love of nature and reminding us that we are animals living with nature in an interplay of life. The movements exemplify the strength of animals and their powers of self-defense. Each of the forms has a martial application.

We are all part of the great universal soup,
all relating to our ever-changing environment,
all part of one system of life on earth breathing together.

Legend says Chang San Feng was born on the revered Wudang Mountain at the end of the Sung Dynasty in April of 1247. His name means three mountain peaks because he lived on three of the sacred mountains of China. He lived through the Mongol period of the Yuan Dynasty and into the Ming dynasty, a period of more than 200 years. The great warrior, Chang, was a monk-scholar sought by emperors for his service. He was famous for evading them. For ten years he resided at the Shaolin Temple where he mastered the martial arts, meditation, and was known as a medical practitioner. He created Tai Chi Chuan, the Supreme Ultimate Fist, a practice of thirteen martial forms done slowly and continuously. He oriented the forms to the Ba Gua, the Eight Directions, and infused them with Taoist philosophy.

Tai Chi is like dancing with the stars and being able to feel the moving molecules of medicine flow through your body at the same time. It is a joyful celebration of life and the life force energy of your breathing body. The whole body is physically engaged. When performed in a group you feel in tune with each other. I used to laugh that it was almost as good as sex, but without the complications.

Will you take this dance? Tai Chi provides a daily sanity in an insane world. It gives good health, self-defense, and greater wisdom. Tai chi cleanses, balances, and strengthens the body. It keeps the mind sharp. It restores the sweet spirit of All is Well! or Haola! You can do it by yourself and never be alone. You can do it with a group, and be part of a Tai Chi family, a rich community cultivating the simple compassion of moving together for health, harmony, and self-defense.

Practice Nine:
Opening Form or
Preparation Stance

Connecting to Earth and Heaven, we allow those energies
to move through us without effort. Stand in Wuji for
a few moments and feel the movement in the stillness.
In Preparation Stance, the posture of Wuji becomes Tai
Chi. In this movement, the stillness of Simple Standing
and the Sinking Down into earth energy, turns into an
upward movement. As if a ball of energy is lifting them,
the arms rise up together. Your palms face the earth. Your
wrists feel as if they are being pulled up to heaven like
they are attached to puppet strings. At their height, the
ball of energy is released to heaven like a prayer. As the
wrists slowly drop down, the fingers follow. As the arms
slowly descend, the heavenly energy is brought down. It
moves through the upper dan tien in the head. The palms
face the earth as your hands lower to either in front of
the middle dan tien at the heart or all the way down to
below the lower dan tien through the Sea of Qi. As you
repeat this movement you can feel the Qi rise and sink
and fill the body and energy centers. One teacher told me
that a person could get Tai Chi benefits from just doing
Opening Form. It contains all there is to know; the rest
of the forms are variations.

Principles of Tai Chi

(which may apply to some forms of Qigong)

Most people who have seen Tai Chi are captured with its graceful movements. But why does it look so graceful? The slow movements are ever changing yet imbued with the consistency of evenness. For me Tai Chi Chuan is a beautiful art form of slow choreography that helps me balance my body, my mind, and my attitude with its even tempo of continuous movement coordinated with my breath in a moving meditation.

Attention and concentration are centered and at ease, like a hawk trying to catch a rabbit or a cat waiting for a mouse. There's no visible exertion in the movements. The forms are martial, but the force is hidden as intrinsic or stored energy. The outer appearance is soft and the inner force is firm. Movements which are also called forms, comprise the yin/yang energy exchange shifting one into the other. Yin/yang is expressed with the inhale and exhale, the solid and empty, the expansion and contraction. The strike turns into the yin recoil which empowers another yang extension. If you over extend you will collapse. All movements are contained by being rooted and in balance.

The evenness of Tai Chi is seen in the consistent flow of the movements. The graceful appearance is maintained because the knees are slightly bent, the eyes are focused on the horizon or looking at the hands. The body stays at the same level with a few exceptions like Snake Creeps Down or Reach for the Needle at the Bottom of the Sea.

Tai Chi teaches greater control of our movements because they are performed with slowness. When we speed up the forms, they are more accurate. It is the same for a pianist, who practices slowly until her fingers are trained in accuracy. Then she can speed up to the desired rhythm.

Softness is attained by going slowly and calmly. Rooted in balance and deep breathing, softness helps us relax. When we are relaxed the circulation is unimpeded, blood and lymph flow, and nerves relax. Any tension in the body reduces energy flow. The Qi flows through the meridians unobstructed. We can take time to stretch out without injury and increase the suppleness of our body.

> The 10,000 creatures and all plants and trees
> are supple and soft in life,
> but brittle and dry in death.
> Truly, to be stiff and hard is the way of death.
> To be soft and supple is the way of life.
> Tao Teh Ching

Five Essential Qualities

Tai Chi exemplifies the Five Qualities of slowness, evenness, calmness, clarity, and balance. The slow and even expression of gathering in and sending out coordinates with the breath and Qi flow. The expanding Qi and the contracting Qi connect with the breathing power of the whole body. Each form and movement connect to the next, evenly and continuously.

Slowness brings an attitude of calmness and tranquility and helps the Qi flow smoothly. It also allows the clarity of each movement to be fully expressed. The powerful spiral energy of the Qi is felt coming up from the earth through the feet. It moves into the lower dan tien, then moves into the arms and hands. The hands become the final expression of the movement. If it is a kick the expression is finalized through the foot. Every movement comes from our center, which is connected to heaven and earth.

Clarity is necessary in moving from one movement to the next. The practitioner finds the final expression of the movement in the extremities of the hands then returns the energy to the lower dan tien. Then the even flow of Qi can be gathered and expanded. Clarity of expression can be seen in the turn of the wrist, the shape of the arm and the alignment of the body. Maintaining the shape of the forms allows Qi to flow without blockage and gives each movement power. The mind leads and the body responds.

The continuous movements of the Tai Chi forms require endurance for five to twenty minutes. Each movement has a martial application. Tai Chi forms are much longer sequences than Qigong forms. Tai Chi is like having many Qigong forms strung together in an even, continuous flow.

Because the practitioner must remember 24 to 108 movements, Tai Chi is a practice in cognitive therapy. The transitions between the movements can be challenging, often taking years of practice and study.

Balance is one of the greatest benefits of Tai Chi practice. When you know where your center of gravity is located, you are in balance. We have a vertical axis that goes through the body and aligns with gravity, called the centerline. The centerline follows our shifts in weight. If we extend too far over and beyond the centerline, we lose our balance and topple. Balance is maintained by being aware of the yin/yang energy as it moves between solid and empty steps. The solid foot is the weight-bearing foot. In a continuous flow, the root of balance moves from the solid yin foot to the empty yang foot. Balance requires being in awareness of our axis and moving with the centerline of gravity. We are rooted while in motion and in control of our balance.

Essential Qualities of Tai Chi are Balance, Evenness, Calmness, Clarity and Slowness.

Spiral Energy

With the axis established, the circular forms of Tai Chi tap into a spiraling energy. Power is expressed through a spiraling movement. This movement extends and unfolds from the centerline to the edge of power. This edge of power is the limit of our ability to balance. We can only go so far out before we must return to the center. The energy force loops back to return to the center. This is sometimes called recoil power. This is the power of a coiled snake.

Spiral energy can contract or expand. Think of skaters performing "crack the whip." The skaters hold hands, making a line from the center of the circle out to the edge of the circle. The person in the center of the circle is the anchor. The anchor moves very little yet has the power to send a ripple down the line of skaters. The skater on the outside receives the energy and moves the fastest, sometimes flying off the end of the whip. In this case the energy moves from the center to the outside. Energy moves in spirals whether it is expanding or contracting.

Tai Chi Chuan is the great dance of moving energy. Energy comes in packets of yin/yang, on/off, positive force/negative force in motion. In Tai Chi practice we learn to keep our balance while moving. Tai Chi is the art of staying centered in the midst of change.

> ## A calm serene energy of peace develops. It echoes the name, Tai Chi, "Peaceful Energy."

Basic Principles

Personal Daily Practice

In order to receive the rewards of Qi medicine, a daily practice is advised. It is a discipline. Daily practice maintains good health by running a check-up through the meridian system, aligning the Fields of Cinnabar, organ washing and tendon changing. However, practicing the traditional standards like Ba Duan Jing, Yi Jin Jing, or the Taoist Walking Circle are essential to a classic Qigong.

Tai Chi and Qigong Body Positions and Stances

There are many varieties of Tai Chi Chuan and many opinions about the correct way to hold the body. "That's not how we do it in OUR form!" is a common response when sharing information between practitioners. Is the body held straight in alignment with the Thrusting Channel or is there a great curve in the torso as well as the arms and legs?

In my tradition the body is held in alignment with the axis, and we don't lean. In this way the body can be relaxed, and the Qi can flow. The shoulders relax over the hips. The elbows are slightly bent and relaxed. The wrists are rarely bent allowing Qi to move through to the hands except for palm strikes when Qi is expressed through the palm.

Foot positioning also varies. Some schools put the whole foot down at once. Others step with the toes first and then put the heel down, but I prefer placing the heel down first in most cases.

The classic horse stance is a Qigong standing position where the feet are placed wider than the shoulders. The knees are bent up to a 90-degree angle, and the back is straight. This stance builds strength in the thighs. The arms are usually held in a Universal Post or "hug a tree" position.

In the modified horse stance, the feet are shoulder width apart and parallel. The toes point in the same direction as the knees. The knees are bent, but not beyond the toes. This stance is used in opening and closing the Tai Chi form. It is when we are coming from and returning to Wuji, the only double weighted position in the form. Rarely is the weight evenly distributed. We are always shifting our weight for greater agility.

The bow stance is used in most Tai Chi moves, such as Combing the Horses Mane, Grasping the Sparrows Tail, or when changing direction. This is the stable stance you take while shooting an arrow from a bow, not on a horse but on the ground. The weighted back foot is at 45 degrees, the front empty foot is pointing straight ahead. The eyes look in the same direction as the forward toe, aligned with the target.

Generally, the direction of the body, the knees, hips, and shoulders are in line with the weighted foot. The orientation of the body changes with the weight shift as it is led by the lower dan tien.

In bow stance there is a space of at least one fist width down the center line between the feet. This is called, "keeping a path between your legs." Keeping a wide path between the legs provides for greater stability and maneuverability.

Movement

In Tai Chi the whole body shifts in the direction the weight goes. The knee is never beyond the toe. When the empty foot steps out, the body weight gradually shifts in the direction the toe points. The empty side becomes the solid position. As you step out with your empty foot, the toe usually points in the new direction, which is often 90-degrees. We are always in relationship to the Eight Directions. If you are facing north and want to go west, your left foot steps back with the toe pointing west. The right heel or toe moves to create the 45-degree angle of a bow stance for stability. Positions shift constantly as the direction of movement changes and the feet are adjusting into and out of the Bow stance.

Coming from a bow stance, you enter a Cat Stance by bringing the forward foot into an empty position with about 10% of its weight on the ball of the foot. It rests in line with the instep of the other 90% weighted foot. This weight bearing stance is good for building muscle strength in the legs and bone density. The body is in position to kick without losing balance. The ball of the foot is used as a striking surface, like there is a fist in your foot.

When one foot steps behind the stationary leg and locks the knee against the outer calf of the stationary leg for support, it is called a twisted stance. The forward leg is kept fairly straight with the knee over the toe, but not beyond it. This is the stance for Embrace the Tiger or Scissor Block. You can lower the body and maintain stability.

Hands, Arms, and Holding the Qi Ball

Throughout the forms the hands change from an open palm to a fist and sometimes an Eagle's Beak. The Eagle's Beak or Mantis Hand gathers up energy, with the fingers together, pointing down to the earth, and the wrist bent up towards heaven. The high bend of the wrist is seen as a weapon like a fist or an elbow. It is also used as a hook to trap, block and parry an opponent.

When the arm moves into a blocking position, protecting the body or head from attack, the wrist naturally rotates to palm out which offers the strong arm bone, on the little finger side of the arm, to receive the blow. This way the palm is out and ready for a grab, and a return to the center of power in the lower dan tien. Movement originates from the feet, is empowered by the lower dan tien, and finds its final expression through the rotation of the wrist and palm.

> # The Palms often connect energetically through the Lao Gong points forming a Qi Ball of energy

The palms often connect energetically through the Lao Gong points, located in the center of the palms. This forms a Qi ball of energy. Even though the hands are held at various distances from each other, when the Lao Gong are aligned, the Qi ball of energy can morphs to stretch and expand or gather and condense. The descending hand drops under the lower dan tien, connecting to the Sea of Qi to receive power through this "bank account of Qi," sending it in the desired direction of final expression.

Practice Ten:
Pull Silk or Silk Reeling

Begin with your feet shoulder width apart. Hold a ball of Qi with your left hand on top, in front of the middle dan tien, and your right hand below your lower dan tien. The top left hand pushes down the body, pushing out impurities. The bottom right hand rises up on the outside of the left hand. The two hands relate to each other, as if pushing down one hand causes the rising of the other. Look into the palm of the hand that is rising. The bottom wrist turns so the palm moves from pushing down to gathering Qi under the lower dan tien. The upper wrist turns to face the other hand to form a Qi ball. The pulling silk practice continues pressing down and rising up in continuous movement. The breath follows only one hand, i.e. exhale as the right hand descends and inhale as it rises. Sifu Nam Singh said the movement was like an old taffy making machine as it moves the strands in continuous flow.

Pulling silk from a cocoon maintains the principle of evenness, not too tight, not too loose, just the right amount of tension.

Pulling Silk is a good preliminary practice
to Wave Hands Like Clouds

Practice Eleven:
Wave Hands Like Clouds

Wave Hands Like Clouds is a movement in Tai Chi forms, usually repeated three times. It can also be a Qigong practice and repeated many times. It lends itself to group practice and can be done in a circle. Energy is moved up through the body and then out to the sides as your arms make big circles. You step sideways like a crab. The waist turns side to center and then to the other side. The arms are always in front of the centerline. As a martial practice, the arms move up to block an attack and then move out to divert it. As a meditation practice you can feel the energy in your emotional gut-brain and name the deep feelings that come up to be transformed by your compassionate heart.

From a Simple Standing position with both hands under the lower dan tien or Sea of Qi, take a breath. On the next inhale, as you raise your right hand up through the lower dan tien to the middle dan tien, be aware of the energy rising. Your arm is slightly curved but not bent. If your elbow is too bent, the Qi will be blocked and not flow, like a bend in a hose slows the flow of water. Look into your right palm. Then turning the upper body to the right, step out to the side with the left foot. The left foot and right hand are extended on a diagonal. By rotating the wrist and letting the palm face out, simply let the energy in your palm go and release. Then let your arm descend. Simultaneously move the weight to the left. Moving back to center, as the right arm is lowering, the left hand gathers energy from the lower dan tien and rises up to eye level. Turn your body through your waist to the left. Your left wrist turns so that your hand can reaches out as if grasping into the direction you are moving. You can feel the diagonal line from your left hand to your right foot. With your weight on the left foot, your right foot comes in next to your left foot and the left arm descends. Your weight shifts to the right so your left foot can step out to the side again, as the right arm rises. Your eyes follow the hands.

If you are moving in the direction to the left, your right hand lets go and your left hand is grasping. If you are moving to the right, it is opposite. We grasp the new and let go of the old.

As one arm descends, with your palm pressing down towards the earth and circling in to below the lower dan tien, your other hand begins to rise up through your centerline. One arm rises as the other one sinks. You look into the rising palm. You turn the waist as the arms move from side to side. The hands and arms stay in front of the body. As in meditation, energy is constantly rising and falling like clouds that come and go.

Reciprocity

A Relationship of Mutual Benefit

As humans we are born of the earth, which is part of the wonders of the universe we call Heaven. In Qigong we call these the Three Powers: Earth, Heaven, and Humanity. We are a manifestation of earth and heaven. There is an exchange of Heaven and Earth within our Humanity, "The universe is in us, as we are in the universe."

The material elements in our body were created in the super nova blasts of stars. The earth is composed of the elements that came from these stars. All is created by the laws of nature we call physics. We have unfolded the mysteries of light, vibration of wave and particle. We can identify the elements, the building blocks of nature combining, separating, recombining, and changing under pressure. This is the harmony of yin and yang, give and take, cause and effect.

Our mother earth flows through us in the form of food, water, and the air we breathe. We are an integral part of the planet. We perceive and receive the beauty of nature which nurtures our spirit, to remember itself. This consciousness lives in our heart and mind, and it knows what love is. We are aware and feel our connection to all life. It is the Shen spirit that inhabits our body beyond our thoughts and stories.

Yin and Yang in Loving Balance

In Qigong and Tai Chi practice we acknowledge the reciprocity of life-breath energy, as plants and animals constantly exchange the gases that give each life. This yin/yang, inhale/exhale, is part of the one breath of Earth itself. Qi is often called, "life-breath energy." Life is totally interconnected by breath. If we lose the oxygen making plants, we suffocate.

Recently a student suggested I read <u>Braiding Sweetgrass</u>. I found it delightful and similar to my understanding of Taoist philosophy. The author, Robin Wall Kimmerer, teaches that all of our flourishing is mutual. As a Ph.D. botanist and Native American, she blends the cultural and spiritual respect that indigenous people have to earth, with modern science. She teaches the power of reciprocity as the native American Indians practiced it. "The elders taught that the relationship between plants and humans must be one of balance. People can take too much and exceed the capacity of the plants to share again." The harvesters never take more than half, and they never take the first patch they find, to ensure its survival. "The grass gives its fragrant self to us and we receive it with gratitude. In return, through the very act of accepting the gift, the pickers open some space, let the light come in and with a gentle tug bestir the dormant buds that make new grass. Reciprocity is a matter of keeping the gift in motion through self-perpetuating cycles of giving and receiving." Ms. Kimmerer's studies show that harvesting is an integral aspect of survival. When the sweetgrass is not harvested, it gets crowded and dies.

The Ants and the Peony

Many years ago, I became aware of the reciprocity of nature in my own back yard. I was happy to see so many buds on my favorite peony plant. As I examined the plant closely, I was dismayed to find the buds were covered with ants! I was horrified and perplexed because I had made a commitment to never again use poisons to kill bugs. After all, to kill a bug is the same poison that would kill a person and why would I want to promote those kinds of substances on the earth? I realized we have to find a better way to rid ourselves of pests without ultimately hurting ourselves. So how would I get rid of these ants without using some terrible product?

When I asked a botanist friend of mine what to do, she assured me that in fact the peonies depend on the ants to help open them. People who raise peonies believe that the nectar the peonies produce lures the ants so that they will come and do their ant dance atop the buds and help them open. Google sites debate this, as peonies do open without ants; however, research substantiates that large peonies may use ants to open and that ants also fight off other dangerous insects. The folklore tradition leaves the ants alone to do their ancient work.

After all, we are part of this wonderful natural interconnection. We breathe with the trees, and all the green things of the earth, in much the same way. They give us the oxygen we need, and we exhale our carbon dioxide that the plants need to exist. We are a breathing, dancing, oneness. We live in an eco-system where we all rely on each other.

I am reminded to trust the universal unfolding. I had a new appreciation of the depth of what the "Trust Your Intuition" magnet on my refrigerator meant. The evolutionary process has given us an inter-dependence for our survival. Sometimes we are the ant, driven to find the peony so we can dance to the fragrance of our bliss. Sometimes we are the peony, and we have to be patient until the ant finds us, so we can open to our beauty.

SEVEN

Health and Healing

Ni hao ma? How are you?

In China, as in many countries, a common greeting is "Ni hao ma?" It simply means, How are you? At formal dinners or in a bar, when a toast is given, we often say, "To your health!"

> **Our health is the center of our life. It determines what we can or cannot do.**

Natural health and healing are the main reasons we practice Qigong and Tai Chi. In order to have a better quality of life, we massage and move every tissue, organ, and joint to refresh and restore our body to its natural state of health.

Our body is built on millions of years of evolving DNA, the magical recipe for life. Life force energy is programmed for survival. The body heals and restores itself as long as it is able. The mind-body treatments of Qigong support our natural ability to stay healthy, and to heal, by strengthening our immune system. They increase our balance and flexibility and repair our injuries.

Like everything in nature, we are in constant change from birth, through our maturity, to our inevitable death. Through the process of evolution, we are all part of the great life experiment on earth. We cycle and process our Qi through our many internal systems. From our first breath, we are breathing with the plants and trees that provide the oxygen needed by every cell of our body. Our body, like the earth, contains the elements created in the stars. We are all intimately connected through ever-changing matter and energy. Through gentle movement and conscious breathing, Qigong and Tai Chi work with nature and promise a longer, healthier, happier life

Cycles of Life

Jing and Health

The life we are given comes from our parents and is known as our Jing energy. Throughout our life, what we do with our Jing determines the state of our health. When we use up our Jing, we die. Each stage from infancy to old age develops different qualities of advancement and decline. As they move down the river of life, the adept goes with the flow. They know how to miss the boulders and avoid injury. With awareness, we adapt and are appropriate to our body and environment and avoid illness and injury. The purpose of our practice is to live fully in the given moment to the best of our ability.

Our health depends on the choices we make that support what we've been given by our ancestors. When you take care of what you've got you can go further. Just like a car, if you don't change the oil and get a tune up, you can ruin the engine. We are co-creators of our health. We may inherit our material body from our ancestors, but we have choices in what we do with it. What happens to us by chance also plays a role.

Even when we are vigilant about good health, it doesn't guarantee a longer life. There are mysterious factors beyond our control, such as having clean water, clean air, fertile soil, and a low stress lifestyle. Our health is influenced by the period of history in which we live; wars, famine, and displacement take their toll. Accidents which cause injury also have a role in our health and well-being.

I define health as the sum of how our body, mind, and spirit are doing at any given moment. When evaluating our health, TCM looks at the personal quality and various characteristics of our whole being, including our attitude. According to the Five Element Theory, our condition or type may be characterized as damp, hot, cool, dry, or wind. These characteristics are called our "climate." The practitioners of TCM find patterns of disharmony and seek to re-balance the body. Qigong, acupuncture, and herbs are used to reharmonize and stimulate energy flow, to decrease stagnation and disease, and to balance yin/yang energy.

Everyone Dies

My mother died at 63 of breast and bone cancer. Her mother died at 44. Mom chose two paths for her treatment. She struggled with all the modern treatments of radical surgery, chemotherapy, and radiation for a couple of years after her diagnosis. She was also involved in a religious group that believed in faith healing.

The whole congregation prayed for her and performed "laying on of hands," to send the power of Jesus to restore her to wholeness. She also fasted and prayed like Jesus in the desert for forty days and forty nights, only drinking water, although she admitted to eating one potato chip because she craved salt.

The laying on of hands my mother received was similar to Qi treatments or Reiki treatments which use natural positive energy to harmonize and heal. Although prayer and energy medicine are known to have great healing possibilities, they didn't save my mother's mortal life.

It was ironic that my father outlived my mother by thirteen years. Mom didn't drink alcohol or smoke, but my father drank alcohol, sometimes heavily. He smoked at least three packs of Pall Mall cigarettes daily and worked as a saw filer in a wood mill for over twenty years breathing iron filings, which resulted in emphysema. He died after a stroke at 81. We each have different propensities for health and illness. Being aware of our particular health issues and how our body works can tip the scale in our favor if we take the measures to support our health and healing.

Taking care of our health is an aspect of chuan, whether we use wholistic (holistic) medicine or allopathic care or both. Chuan is the fist of self-containment we practice in Tai Chi Chuan. It is the quality of taking responsibility for yourself and refusing to be a victim. It is courage in the face of difficulties.

I am old now and more capable in some regards of choosing where and how I place my attention. Yet the energy required for completion of my projects is less. These days I appreciate the Taoist precept, to do less! I am sorting out what I want to leave behind. I'm putting my life in order, leaving my legacy in the form of this book. I'm making space for my old age to be lived with more serenity.

In our modern culture we worship youth and abhor the old. In the West it is acceptable for people to say they are younger than their age. In the East the opposite is true. Being old is revered. In American culture we fear death. It is not part of life as it was in past generations when the old lived at home and died at home. Now we distance ourselves from death by putting the old and frail into nursing homes. We even deny death when we buy meat that is packaged neatly and divorced from the process of slaughtering or butchering. To extend life, we endure great suffering and pain with surgeries, chemo therapies, feeding tubes, and ventilators. Sometimes these conditions are fates worse than death. Death can be a refuge, a relief from suffering.

Traditional Chinese Medicine, TCM

The practices of Traditional Chinese Medicine, including Qigong, Tai Chi Chuan and Taoism are rooted in legends. Ancient legends of China tell of the great shamans who changed the course of the Yellow River to prevent flooding. Shamanic leaders united the people, creating culture. There are stories of wise people and healers who lived in sacred mountains as hermits.

Traditional Chinese Medicine is an ancient system, that originated with the shamans and hermits. It uses herbs, acupuncture, moxibustion, cupping, massage, Qigong movement and rest. Through balancing yin and yang energies harmony is restored. Acupuncturists stimulate various acupuncture points with needles along meridians to treat diseases or simply to rejuvenate the body with a "tune up." TCM also prescribes Qigong practice to stimulate specific meridians and acupressure points. Many TCM doctors are also medical Qigong practitioners who use specific Qigong practices to address health issues.

Acupuncturists are often herbalists who use a variety of Chinese herbs. These herbs have been studied and cultivated for centuries. Sifu Nam Singh took me to some of the herb shops in San Francisco's Chinatown in the late 70's. The pungent smell met us before we entered the front door. I was fascinated by the many jars of medicine, shelf after shelf all the way to the ceiling. These jars contained dried herbs, and berries, seeds and nuts, and sometimes animals, like tiny seahorses. There were big cases of many drawers that held more herbs and potions behind the long counter. Several herbalists, who spoke Cantonese, worked with customers. Prescriptions were read, and the herbalist would pull out drawers, or get on ladders to retrieve jars. They piled the dried ingredients onto a big piece of paper, weighed it and wrapped it up with instructions. Even the food markets had healing herbs and foods like sea weeds, funguses that looked more ominous than edible, and many strange forms of dried bean curd. Sifu himself was an herbalist and worked in Chinatown for several years. He now teaches medicinal cooking using herbs and food.

Moxibustion is another common treatment in TCM. It is heat therapy made by burning Moxa, the compressed herb mugwort (Artemisia vulgaris). It is burned next to various acupuncture points to stimulate a point and to prevent fainting. Cupping uses glass cups or bamboo jars to create a vacuum suction to stimulate blood flow and control other conditions.

Qigong and Tai Chi are exercises designed to maintain the body at optimal efficiency. They are based on the premise that our body wants to be healthy, and the will to live is very strong when it is supported. When the Qi flow is open, it brings harmony wherever it goes.

Qi Treatment

Our health depends on how we are balancing, what we take in and what we release, how we move and how we relax.

> # Qigong and Tai Chi are treatments that strengthen and cleanse all our systems through gentle movements which keep our fluids flowing.

Qigong and Tai Chi are called "medicine in motion." Primarily this is preventative medicine, but through daily practice the ancient healing arts of Qigong and Tai Chi also heal us when we are sick or injured. Practice integrates the whole body and mind and returns us to good health.

The Power of Relaxation

We learn to relax so the body can come into balance, which requires stillness. Stillness allows Qi to flow. That is why Wuji is the beginning of most Qigong forms. After we come into stillness, we bring our mind's attention to our breath. Our breath is a tool we use to help us relax. We listen to our body in its present state, using our will in a spacious, loving way. We direct Qi flow with our breath to loosen the tight, stuck places. We breathe into any painful places to relieve the pain and allow restoration. As we draw the inhale through the nostrils, like "smelling a rose," the breath is even and slow. The exhale is even and slow, like "blowing on a flute." When we are cleansing, we breathe out through the mouth with a long exhale to release pain and tightness. In Qigong we relax and move our body in coordination with our breath.

Power of Calmness and the Vagus Nerve

One main reason we concentrate on deep breathing in Qigong is to stimulate the vagus nerve. The vagus nerve is the biggest nerve in the body. It is sometimes called the wandering nerve. It runs from the brain through the face, thorax, and abdomen. It provides visceral sensation to the heart, the abdominal viscera, taste sensations in the mouth. It affects a majority of muscles, the immune system, and the parasympathetic nervous system. About 80% of the vagus nerve sends sensory information back to the brain about the body's organs. Visceral feelings and gut instincts are emotional intuitions transferred to the brain by the vagus nerve. These gut feelings have been linked to altering moods, fears, and anxieties. This mind-body feed-back loop gives us the reactions of fight and flight or rest and digest.

The "gut brain," also called ENS enteric nervous system is two thin layers of more than 100 million nerve cells lining your gastrointestinal tract from your esophagus to your rectum. Many health issues are related to a healthy digestive system. Healthy microbes in your digestive system are essential for the health both physically and mentally. The gut and its microbes control inflammation and make many different compounds that can affect brain health. These can control anxiety, stress, and depression.

A healthy vagus nerve is stimulated with a few deep breaths that include long exhales. About five long exhales can create a state of inner calm and promote healing. When the vagus nerve is stimulated in this way the heart rate slows, blood pressure is lowered, and inflammation and depression is reduced.

Practice Twelve:
Stand Like a Mountain

Use Wuji and Simple Standing posture for five minutes or more with the following stillness meditation:

Stand like a mountain unmoving,
though the seasons change,
the mountain remains,
the image of stillness.

Think of yourself as a mountain. Imagine how you are connected deep into the earth and soaring high into the sky. Notice your massiveness and majesty, your stable grounding. Imagine how you lie in stillness beneath the sky as day changes into night and returns to day. Feel the clouds and wind moving across your body. The clouds may cover your body, but you remain beneath unchanged. Imagine the vegetation and animals you may support. Feel the rays of the sun, warming your surface. Imagine the seasons as one changes into the next. Let each season come and go: the warmth of summer, the colors of fall, the cold winter. Feel the blanket of snow melting into spring and the newness of life as wild flowers adorn your body. The mountain remains in stillness with all the changes it experiences.

Rest

The rejuvenation of our body, and its detoxification, is mostly done when we are asleep. When we sleep, the parasympathetic nervous system, which controls our organs, can fully operate without the distraction of our sensory responses. During sleep our body restores itself by cleaning out waste products. For example, when we sleep more blood flows to the liver and is cleansed. There is new evidence that getting enough sleep may help prevent Alzheimer's disease because the brain has a chance to clean out the substances that can cause Alzheimer's. Brain waves are slower when we sleep, and our muscles relax and repair. The brain reviews complex stimuli and uses this information to make more informed decisions when we awake. The notion of sleeping on a big decision is a good idea. In Qigong and Tai Chi meditation practice we create a healing condition similar to sleep except that we maintain consciousness and can direct the mind and body.

Times and places of stillness and relaxation are often prescribed by doctors because they know stress is a major contributor to disease. The stillness of Wuji allows the mind to settle down from the chaos of stories the mind can create. The mind is brought into the service of the body, a reversal from the norm.

Food and Herbs

A common greeting in China:
Ni chi fan le ma, or Did you eat?

Traditional Chinese Medicine originated with hermits who created Qigong practices. They had great understanding of herbs and their properties for healing. In TCM it is common to think of food as medicine. We receive Qi from the Qi of what we eat. Other than most medicinal foods which are dried, fresh food has more nourishing Qi: The fresher the better. That's why growing your own food can be so beneficial.

Everyone has slightly different needs, so we learn overtime what is good for us, and what doesn't agree with our particular system. Several Tai Chi masters I've talked with, advise eating early in the morning, usually including a little pickle which helps create an alkaline base in our system. The middle of the day is the main meal, and then a smaller meal is eaten at the end of the day. Alkaline foods like leafy greens and most vegetables support the body's health. Acid foods like sugar, other carbohydrates, and red or processed meats create inflammation and are more difficult to digest. Interestingly, lemons and cider vinegar have an alkalizing effect on the body even though they are acids. They are excellent for cleansing the body and reducing inflammation. A little lemon in your tea is a good practice!

Healing Disease

Qigong and Tai Chi are sometimes called "medicine in motion." First, in stillness, we find our center like the axis of the earth. Then we move around it, so we are relaxing into our center and expanding from our center. The gentle circles loosen the joints, and massage the muscles, organs, and tissues of the body.

Stagnation of Qi causes putrefaction like water that doesn't move. Movement pushes out stale energy, impurities, and debris. Pathogens are released and can be expelled. We send healing rejuvenating Qi to all parts of our body. When we have an injury, we can be afraid to move. In order to keep moving, we have to keep moving. In soft persistence there is strength.

Several of my students with cancer claim their daily practice of the PYNK Qigong form kept their cancer in remission. Students with Parkinson's disease have improved their balance and increase the quality of their life. People with stress disorders and mental illness calm down and find clarity. Many people are able to reduce their pharmaceuticals. Bone density increases, blood pressure lowers, and people find better balance physically and emotionally.

Most students find they are happier and healthier when they practice. After a twenty-minute PYNK Qigong treatment, the whole body feels alert and yet relaxed. The Qi energy is felt as a tingling, open aliveness that permeates the whole body. Most describe a warm glow and a natural state of contentment and well-being.

Healing Injury

I hurt my shoulder working with developmentally challenged patients at the State Hospital before I began a Tai Chi practice. The pain was almost unbearable. My employer put me on disability and sent me to a physical therapist who put me on a routine of traction.

While I was on his therapy table, I also had to endure the humiliation of him massaging my breast, as if it were part of my therapy. I was frozen in disbelief. I naively thought this man, as a doctor, wouldn't do anything inappropriate. I didn't say anything, but I never went back, and the incident made my pain worse.

It wasn't until I started taking Tai Chi class that the old scar tissue in my shoulder loosened up and I could gain the range of motion I had lost. The old memory came back too, and I healed from the humiliation I felt. Tai Chi practice and my training at PAWMA Camp had taught me to be alert, trust my intuition, and be ready to act quickly to get out of a bad situation. Martial arts gave me confidence.

When I lived on the farm, I hurt my back hauling 80-pound feed bags and hay bales. My general practitioner prescribed painkillers and muscle relaxers, but I didn't like the side effects and they didn't always work. Tai Chi helped me relax and be more flexible. I would get better and then I'd do too much and reinjure myself. It took a long time for me to learn to do less and let myself heal. I learned to appreciate the messages my body gave me and listened.

The range of motion exercises in Qigong helped me strengthen my joints and realign my body. I also used Lian Gong as taught by Wen Mai Yu. Lian Gong alleviates pain stiffness and heals injuries with specific gentle Qigong stretches and Qi treatments. Qigong feeds our tissues and promotes healing with nutrients and increased blood circulation. Often the injured area is rested, while the joints on either side of the injury are gently engaged to promote circulation.

Rest, Mantras, and Movement

I started taking better care of myself. I would ask for help and use better body mechanics when I had to move something heavy. If I was feeling soreness or tension, I would lie down. I would send healing Qi into the injured area and relax deeply. This took a lot of patience. I had to learn to wait and give my body time to heal. When the inflammation decreased, with easy ROM (range of motion) massaging circles, I could start rebuilding my strength and flexibility.

I would also repeat mantras. My favorite mantra for healing the lower back pain came from the intuitive healer Louise Hay. I repeat it over and over and feel a powerful healing energy fill my whole being.

"I trust the universe, life itself supports me."

The combination of rest, mantras, and movement helped me heal and strengthen. I learned to make space for change and cultivate the yin of emptiness, which is Wuji. Somewhere I found a quote that I wrote down and put on the wall next to my mirror that help me understand the power of Wuji.

"Meditation is to rest undistractedly
in the immediate present.
Return to the present.
Return to the unchanging heart of open compassion."

For healing to take place we may be required to look deeper than our physical body. Many illnesses and injuries are caused by emotional trauma. Physical healing often happens when emotional problems are resolved. We may also need to tenderly examine the development of our consciousness and our conditioned behavior to find the roots of an illness. With Wuji practice and stillness our feelings and needs are often more clearly revealed. Sometimes it takes a guide or counselor to help us sort through the entanglements of our emotions and find a way to heal. Healing is an integration of mind, body, and spirit.

Life Force Energy

Qigong is translated as "breath work" or "energy practice." Breath is the essence of life. Our first breath announces our presence to the world and our last breath marks our death. Working with breath energy is the root of meditation practice. When we concentrate on our breath, we both calm and boost our energy. We can use our breath to change our physiology. Inhale and exhale have a receiving and sending aspect that can be used to direct Qi. We can live several days without food and water, but only a few minutes without breath.

Where does breath come from?

Our breath connects us to all life. All the plants and animals on this earth breathe together. We are dependent on plants and their process of photosynthesis which provides the oxygen we need. Photosynthesis started about 2.4 billion years ago when the biological phenomenon of oxidation began. As animals, we breathe with the plants in an exchange of gases. We inhale the oxygen produced from the plants; and in return, we exhale carbon dioxide which the plants take in for photosynthesis. This exchange is known in Qigong as life breath energy.

The Qi character, as shown in chapter one, translates as breath. It depicts a pot with rice cooking symbolizing the nourishing power of Qi. The lid of the pot is lifted because the steam is rising, which indicates the moving power of Qi.

There are many kinds of Qi energy as discussed earlier. The primal Qi is the stuff like quanta that makes up everything. It is a balance of yin and yang in constant exchange. When the Qi condenses it makes form, when it disperses it returns to energy. It is like the interchange of matter and energy in the study of physics. Qi that runs through the meridians of our body is called Meridian Qi. Opening the flow of Qi through the meridians is a primary practice in Qigong.

Harmonize the Qi

Tai Chi and Qigong practices harmonize the flow of Qi through our bodies in continuous and changing patterns. Yin becomes yang, and yang becomes yin in cycles. The pair of opposites intrinsically depend upon one another. Without form, force has no material expression; without force, form is dead. The blend and balance of the macrocosmic energies of force, Qi, and form, Li, manifest through the microcosmic energies of Qi and Jing in our body respectively. Li is the physical form and pattern for the behavior of Qi.

Our arteries are the form through which blood is carried. Our blood delivers oxygen, breath or Qi force, to every cell of our body. When our arteries become clogged the heart must work harder to push blood through our veins. Qigong and Tai Chi practice help the heart circulate blood and open its passages. Closed and stagnant places (yin) are opened and cleansed through movement (yang).

Inner Healer

Trust your Intuition

When we begin the Tai Chi form, we bow in with the hand mudra of the Chain Link of Grace. This is a hand position made by combining the right fist, representing the boxer and yang active side, together with the yin left hand that covers the fist. The left hand represents the scholar or inner teacher. We think before we act. What is this inner teacher? How does it work?

Intuition is immediate cognition based on an inner knowing. When we feel something is wrong with our body, mind, or spirit, we use our intuition. We attend to the feeling, and compare it to the knowledge we have gained about our body from previous experience. Then we can take the action that is appropriate. Listening to our body and using our intuition to give ourselves some tender loving care can help heal and prevent disease.

At the martial arts camp, Cynthia Hale, a karate black belt, taught that our reaction to violence must be immediate. You have to trust your intuition. She said, to prevent rape, women had to move away from trouble or fight back. OK, I thought, but how can I fight a man who is inherently stronger than I am? Cynthia taught self-defense techniques to neutralize an attacker: knee jab to the groin, punch to the Adam's Apple, shove his nose through his brain, poke him in the eye. I didn't want to even think about doing any of those things. Most of us have been trained to be nice, to be ladylike, and to placate men. When we trained to protect ourselves, this conditioning had to be overcome. Through Tai Chi Chuan we become more aware of our surroundings. We learn to quickly recognize danger and rely on innate instincts to get us out of trouble.

Using our Mind to Heal

Our mind is a powerful instrument. How we use it greatly determines our health and well-being. Most of us have a fear of illness and death. When we are diagnosed with an illness, our fears cause stress and further inhibit the body from natural healing. We sometimes condemn ourselves for getting sick. By releasing our fears and judgments, we can make space for change, to get beyond our fear and denial. By examining our thoughts and reframing them we can choose a thought that is more conducive to healing. When we meditate, we softly notice the negative judgments against ourselves and release them.

In Qigong we work with several principles for healing. First is the principle, "what you cultivate grows," which includes, "what you resist persists." Where we put our attention creates more neural synapse connections in the brain and strengthens that pathway. If we are thinking about stressful things, it will likely cause more stress and disease. If you cultivate physical practice, you become stronger physically. If you plant a seed, give it water and nurture it, it becomes a plant.

> # Where the mind goes,
> # the Qi follows.
> # Where the Qi goes,
> # the blood follows.

As in Wuji, Simple Standing practice Qigong practice helps us clear our mind of distracting thoughts. We open the body to the power of earth and heaven and use our breath to support the natural flow of healing energies. We send healing Qi into painful or tight places, whether they are physical, mental, or emotional. Making space for change allows our natural harmony to return. The Qi or breath energy is sent into the afflicted places with the relaxed exhale. Visualizing ourselves whole and well creates a positive image in our brain, which promotes better health.

Wisdom Healing Qigong

Grand Master Pang Ming MD founded the largest Qigong hospital near Beijing in 1980, called Huaxia Zhineng Qigong Center. It was closed by the Chinese government partly due to the trouble caused by the Fulan Gong cult. However, according to my teacher, Ming Tong Gu, in its existence of 25 years, the center treated more than 200,000 patients with 185 different diseases and achieved an overall success rate of 95%. One of Dr. Pang's students,

Luke Chan, brought the practice of Wisdom Healing Qigong to the USA. His book, <u>101 Miracles of Natural Healing</u>, tells the stories of 101 of Dr. Pang's patients who described being healed from cancer, diabetes, heart disease, severe depression, lupus, and many other chronic illnesses. The patients actively engaged in their healing. Although the Qigong was simple, they spent hours in mind–body practice every day. I was fortunate to be able to study with Dr. Pang's student Master Ming Tung Gu, and I learned Wisdom Healing Qigong which is based on Dr. Pang's methods. During the teacher training program, I experienced a profound power in the Qi field. It was like a silent hum in the air that everyone could hear and access to heal.

The training was held in the mountains of Santa Cruz at a Buddhist retreat center. It was a wooded area with many cabins, a big kitchen, a conference hall and temple. It was my job to start the morning fires in the big stove in the kitchen about 6:00 AM. It was sometimes a struggle, as I stayed up to the closing of the evening events and had to gather my own kindling from the forest floor to get the logs started. It was very cold in the mornings and people were looking to get warmed up. They gathered at the big stove drinking their tea and coffee before breakfast. I took my duty seriously and felt I helped contribute to the good Qi field.

Ming Tong was charismatic and created a Qi field that reminded me of the evangelical tent meetings my mother took me to as a child. The atmosphere was expectant, open, and creative. In the early morning we would practice a beginning form in the Wisdom Healing Qigong known as Lift Qi Up and Pour Qi Down, which is done standing in one place.

Ming Tong Gu had us memorize Dr. Pang's Eight Verses to create a Qi field. You can use these eight verses to create a powerful Qi field when practicing by yourself or with others.

Practice Thirteen:
Eight Verses of Dr. Pang

1. **Head touches the sky feet stand on earth.** The visualization is feet plunging deep into the earth all the way to the other side of space, open all gates: crown of the head, feet, hands, and the gate of life.

2. **Body relaxes and mind expands.** With the entire body relaxed, allow the mind-body to expand in the eight directions simultaneously: Entire Qi body expanding and merging into the ocean of Qi.

3. **Be respectful externally and quiet internally.** Respect the omni-presence of the living universe. Mind quieting into the stillness. Enter the Qigong state, beyond the differentiating mind and into ever present grace. Looking inwardly into the center of the brain, the Shenji palace.

4. **Heart is sincere, and appearance is reverent.** Feel the inner smile from the brain into your heart and expanding into the entire body. Feel the deep sincere intention from your heart. Feel the blessing expanding from inside out to all life.

5. **Mind is clear of any thought.** Acknowledging any distracting thoughts or resistance, let them go into the infinity space. Mind is clear like a clear mirror reflecting the space.

6. **Mind expands into the infinite space.** Focus on the vast emptiness of the universe. Allow the expansiveness of the mind to connect to Primal Huan Yin Qi. (Yuan Qi)

7. **Mind's intention embracing entire body inwardly.** Mind is gathering the universal Qi into the inner space of the transparent body.

8. **The entire body is harmonized with Qi.** Feel the warm flow of universal Qi harmonizing the entire body, harmonizing all dimensions deep inside. All is well in the return to oneness.

Master Gu could create an atmosphere that was trance inducing. It was quiet and deep. He included movement, visualization, and sound. He cultivated trust and vulnerability when we were sharing. Master Gu emphasized that the role of the teacher is to inspire and support others, not to fix or find solutions for them. These teachings were very valuable in my own healing practice and helped me be a better teacher.

EIGHT

Ba Gua: Math, Magic, Martial Arts

The Way of Tai Chi Chuan

When I first started to learn the Tai Chi Dragon Tiger Mountain form, I found it difficult to follow even though the movements were done very slowly. Sometimes I'd feel lost, I'd be headed one way and the rest of the class would be moving in the opposite direction. I felt awkward and confused, but I liked the movement and wanted to continue.

Sifu told me to keep track of where you are, it's good to know what direction you're going. He said the Ba Gua provides the map. I learned that every step is oriented to a cardinal direction or a corner. The cardinal directions of South, North, West, and East correspond to Heaven, Earth, Water and Fire. The corners of the Ba Gua, NW,

SW, NE, SE correspond to Mountain, Wind, Thunder, and the Joyous Lake.

Tai Chi is a dance of harmony and oneness expressed through the qualities of yin and yang. The expansion of their possibilities are expressed through the Ba Gua. Ba Gua means eight directions. Within each movement yin and yang are balanced. The soft, still yin provides the open path for strong yang Qi to be demonstrated.

Tai Chi Chuan is translated as Supreme Ultimate Fist and is a powerful martial art. This slow soft Taoist practice is a moving philosophy which develops the quality of "steel in cotton."

The Highest power (te) is not powerful
(not trying to be powerful)
Therefore has true power.
Lower power is always (trying to be) powerful,
Therefore never (attains) power.
Tao Te Ching Chapter 38

When we are in flow with the Tao, in harmony with nature, we have optimal power. This power occurs without effort or individuated ego. Consciousness is focused on the flow of Qi without self-consciousness or distraction.

When I started learning Tai Chi, I was twenty-nine and I was painfully self-conscious. I grew up being teased mercilessly about my small stature. My older half-brother called me "runt" and "bird brain." Tai Chi practice helped me forget about myself. At first it was all I could do to keep up with the flow of the movements, but eventually I got good at it and felt successful. Learning Tai Chi gave me the courage to take on other challenges I had been too afraid to try. I wanted to learn everything I could about this powerful healing art.

Sifu said I should learn about Chinese culture and gave me an old book called <u>Peasant Cults of China</u>. This book was soothing for me because I could relate to the peasant farm life. I was living on twenty acres, raising goats, making cheese and growing my own food.

Roots of a Peasant Culture

For thousands of years the Chinese culture has been based on farming and what is known as the Peasant Cults. In these agrarian communities, people lived in the same place for hundreds of years and developed unique cultures and traditions. As nomadic people began to settle and raise crops and domesticate animals, knowing where and when to plant crops was essential. Before the invention of the written word, they used oral tradition and stories to pass on their information. One of the first yin/yang symbols they used was a mountain with a dark yin side and a bright yang side. As farming people, the path of the sun had meaning for them. They also had to understand the patterns of rainfall, and the direction the wind blew. They were led by shamans and rainmakers; they honored the life-giving "cloud dragon" that nourished their crops. They worked with nature, the

189

sun, the water, and the soil. This is how the traditions of the Five Elements and the Eight Directions began.

Ba Gua and the Eight Directions

The Ba Gua is not simply points on a compass but a philosophy of how creation unfolds. The development of the Ba Gua created a number system that could describe the qualities of Heaven, Earth, and Humanity. The ancient Chinese believed that Creation starts with the Great Tao which is undifferentiated and unknowable. Differentiation started with the Tai Chi. What is one becomes two, the opposing forces of yin and yang. From these forces the rest of creation is formed. The distribution of yin yang energy forms all the various possibilities. Through the Ba Gua, the story of creation and culture came alive.

The structure of the Ba Gua is a circle comprised of eight directions. The circle is divided into dark, yin; and light, yang. The dark yin of the north is Mother Earth. It is dark, cold, night. The general quality of yin contracts. Gravity, balance and stillness are all assigned to yin. The Yang is represented by Father Sky and the south. Yang is an expanding energy. It is bright, light, day. It is the Tao of creation, the expansive energy of the universe, movement and our sense of time as we track the heavenly bodies in the sky.

As you move through the Tai Chi form you are aware of the qualities of the direction you are facing, which adds a sense of poetry and connection to the natural world. The new moon appears in the west. The west represents water and the moon. The moon affects the tides. It is sister to the earth. The east represents fire and the sun. The sun rises in the eastern sky. The sun is the fire of heaven and essential for crops to grow.

The acknowledgment of these celestial bodies that sustain our life on earth was comforting to me. Tai Chi was like a moving prayer of gratitude for my life.

As I shifted from one movement to the next, I noticed constant change was guided by inner consistency. This consistency came from being centered. In the Ba Gua the yin and yang sides of the circle are not a straight line but a curve that implies movement, with the shift of day becoming night, and night becoming day. The constant change of yin becoming yang, and yang turning into yin is often portrayed as two fish swimming in the Tai Chi symbol. Sifu said Tai Chi movements are ever flowing. He said, "Think of a fish swimming. It is constantly moving. A fish doesn't hold still. It is always swimming. That is how Tai Chi form is done. You are always in graceful motion like a fish swimming."

This image of a graceful fish was helpful to me. I would sometimes find myself frozen in confusion. Then I'd remind myself: just keep swimming and go with the flow of the river. I was afraid of change. I wanted to stay safe and have a stable life, yet as a single mom, life was full of unknown and challenging circumstances.

> **With my Tai Chi practice, I learned to flow with the changes and keep my center. Using the qualities of yin yang theory, I felt more at ease in accepting what came and choosing what action to take.**

Tai Chi enacts the principle that in stillness yin/yang come together, in movement they separate. Think of water: when it freezes it is still and solid and when it boils, it is active, turning to steam. Sometimes I still felt frozen in fear. When I didn't deny it and just observed my fears in stillness, I could find a way out based on action not reaction. The frozen fear and anger would turn to steam and give me the power to make successful change.

This power is symbolized by the Chinese character for Qi. As you may remember, the description of the character depicts a pot of boiling water with the lid of the pot lifting as the water turns to forceful steam. The character shows a grain of rice cooking within the pot. This implies that Qi is nourishing.

In stillness we embrace the whole picture of what is going on. When we step back and realize the cause and effect of an action, we can act with empathy. This is the power of Tai Chi. It is the great harmony of opposite poles, like the positive and negative ends of a magnet. As we explored in the first chapter, the practice of Qigong and Tai Chi is based on the principle, "Out of Wuji comes Tai Chi." This phrase translates as, "Out of nothing comes something," or "out of stillness comes movement." The powerful movement we acquire from stillness is based on taking time to see more of the whole picture.

The Ba Gua puts these qualities into a simple form. Something and nothing can be described mathematically as 1 and 0, the binary system of the Ba Gua. A solid line represents yang and the creative power of heaven; an open line or two short lines represent yin and the receptive power of earth.

When the lines are doubled, greater and lesser energies are created that explain various qualities. Greater yang is two solid lines. Greater yin is two sets of open lines. A solid top and an open bottom create lesser yang. An open top and a solid bottom create lesser yin. From these four images another top line is added alternating in yin and yang lines creating the eight trigrams of the Ba Gua.

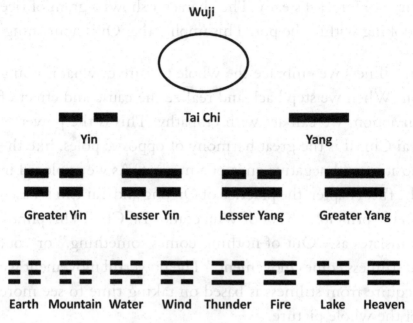

Before Heaven Model

Each trigram is assigned an aspect of nature according to its yin/yang energy. Each line of the trigram represents one of the Three Powers. The bottom line represents earth, the top line heaven, and the middle line stands for humanity.

Fuxi's arrangement is called the Before Heaven model. It is the model we use in Tai Chi. Every movement is oriented to one of the directions. As a map or compass, Heaven is south, and on top, because it represents the southern exposure and the sky. The Earth is north, and on the bottom, the ground, and the dark unknown. We face north to begin our Tai Chi form to honor the earth and acknowledge that we are always facing the unknown.

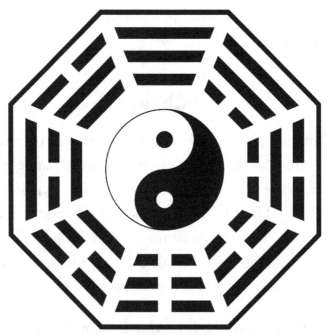

The Ba Gua, Before Heaven diagram.

Heaven is pure yang and Earth is pure yin. Fire in the East and Water in the West are opposite pairs. The cardinal directions and the corners are depicted as family members. The depiction of the youngest son in the northwest is also known as the Mountain. Opposite the Mountain the Joyous Lake represents the youngest daughter in the southeast. Mountains and lakes are both physical structures. The other corners represent forces of nature. In the southwest we have the invisible Wind, the eldest daughter. In the northeast we have the eldest son, which is Thunder. This family order was used by Confucius many centuries after the prehistorical time of Fuxi. In the Before Heaven model, the yin daughters are placed around the yang father, and the yang sons surround the yin mother. The two dots in the Tai Chi symbol represent the yin in the yang, and the yang in the yin.

I Ching

The I Ching is a philosophy of how yin and yang play out their infinite combinations. The eight basic trigrams are combined to form the 64 hexagrams which represent archetypal situations in human life. The I Ching, or Book of Changes, developed over millennia. From its beginning the I Ching has been used as an oracle. People still consult the I Ching to divine their fate and seek knowledge for the best action.

The binary system used in our computers was created thousands of years ago by the Chinese. I Ching is based on the binary system of mathematics of 0 and 1. The German mathematician, Leibniz who studied the I Ching, brought the binary system to western awareness in 1689. He acknowledged Fu Xi in the title of his paper on the new arithmetic.

According to Joseph Needham, the great authority on Chinese science, many mathematical ideas had their origin in China. They include the decimal system, negative numbers, using algebra in geometry, a refined value of *pi,* and "Pascal's Triangle." This was 427 years before Pascal "invented" it! Mathematics is reflected in Chinese Medicine and the theories of Yin/Yang, The Three Powers, The Five Elements, the Eight Directions, and the Thirteen Postures of Tai Chi Chuan. These are the numbers of the Fibonacci sequence which is found throughout the natural world. To generate this sequence, we begin with one. One plus one equal two. One plus two equals three. Two plus three equals five. Continue this pattern by adding the last two numbers to create the next. Five plus three equal eight. Eight plus five equals thirteen.

Many plants exhibit the Fibonacci sequence. We can see that the scales of pinecones are arranged in clockwise and counterclockwise spiraling rows. The number of rows is two adjacent numbers, such as three clockwise, and five counterclockwise. Pineapples spiral their scales in eight clockwise and thirteen counterclockwise rows. Flowers also have this sequence. For example, Irises have three petals, buttercups have five, delphiniums have eight, marigolds have thirteen, asters have twenty-one, and daisies have thirty-four, fifty-five, eighty-four, etc.

The I Ching uses yin yang theory to describe situations like the relationship of land and people. For example, China is a country with lots of land and lots of people. It would be represented by two solid lines, greater yang. Japan has little land and lots of people and would be described as lesser yang. Canada has lots of land but few people and is seen as lesser yin, whereas Iceland has little land and is sparsely populated and is characterized as greater yin.

The After-Heaven Model of the Ba Gua

I was familiar with the Before Heaven model as we use it in Tai Chi to determine the direction of the movements. The After-Heaven model was mysterious to me until Nam

Singh explained that it was how energy flowed through the seasons. It is also used in the art of Feng Shui.

For over a thousand years the Chinese used the Ba Gua of Fuxi. During the Zhou dynasty about 1143 BCE, the Duke of Zhou designed the After-Heaven version of the Ba Gua. It is based on a mysterious order in the I Ching which read like a magical incantation to me. "The ruler comes forth in Chen, (Thunder) to start his creation. He completes everything in Sun (Wind)." This represents spring, the beginning and end of the year in the Chinese calendar. "He manifests things to see one another in Li (Fire) and causes them to serve each other in Kun (Earth). He rejoices in Tui (Lake) and battles in Chien (Heaven). He is comforted and takes rest in Kan (Water) and finishes his work of the year in Ken (Mountain)."

This strange quote in the I Ching gave me a better idea of how energy flowed. The ruler is the will of heaven which comes out of the power of Thunder, the eldest son, as a force that can be compared to mythical qualities of Zeus or Thor. The energy moves clockwise around the circle. It skips the position of Wind, the eldest daughter, which is completion, connecting the old year to the new year in Spring. The energy moves to Fire which represents the life-giving sun at the top of the circle in the place of Summer. It then moves to Late Summer and the position of Earth. The Earth, in the position of mother, is abundant. The naturally harmonious energy of the Tao, together with the energy of the Earth, cause us to serve each other. The cycle continues in Fall, the time of harvest, when we rejoice in the fruits of our labor. The fifth position in the northwest represents Heaven, the position of father.

I believe the phrase "it battles in Heaven" means we struggle to understand the Tao of Heaven and how to live in harmony in this life. The time just before winter is a sacred time in many cultures. The High Holy holidays in Jewish religion end with Yom Kippur, a day of union with God. Halloween, Samhain, and the Day of the Dead, celebrate this time when the veil between heaven and earth is thin and souls return to earth.

Water is represented by the deep, dark winter, when we are "comforted and take rest." Indeed, winter is a time to rest from the year's planting cycle and a time of meditation and contemplation. The work is finished in spring, on the Mountain, and completed with the eldest daughter Wind. To start a new year and a new cycle, it begins again by moving counterclockwise to the eldest son, Thunder.

The After-Heaven model of the Ba Gua was the basis for the development of the Chinese calendar. The directions and seasons of the year also relate to the Five Elements. Spring is associated with east and the element Wood. Summer represents Fire and is in the south. Late Summer represents the element Earth. The Earth element runs through the center of the Ba Gua from the trigram Earth in the southwest to the trigram Mountain in the north east. The element for the west is Metal and the season is fall. The north's element is Water and its season is winter.

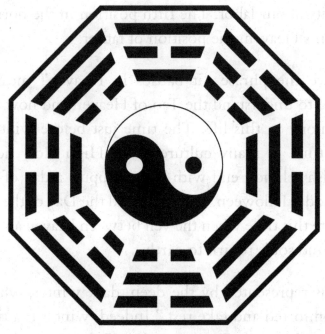

The After Heaven Model

In the Chinese pinyin spelling, which is used currently, Thunder is zhen. The Lake, Tui is spelled dui. Heaven, Chien, is qian. The Mountain, Ken, is gen. Chen, Wind, Sun is xun. Otherwise, it is the same as the Wade-Giles version.

Lo Pan and Feng Shui

The compass of the Ba Gua evolved into an elaborate instrument called the Lo Pan, or Luo Pan which came into use about two thousand years ago. Lo means a net that encompasses everything, pan means utensil or plate. It symbolizes the union of Heaven and Earth and the electromagnetic field that holds all matter together. A real compass with a magnetized needle in the center of this model pointed south, the direction of Heaven.

The mysterious Lo Pan is a very complex system. The concentric circles of information begin with the yin/yang in the center and move out to include the Five Elements, and twelve animal signs of the Chinese zodiac, and their relationship to the Eight Directions.

The Lo Pan is used in the Ba Gua system of Feng Shui arts. Feng Shui has been practiced for thousands of years. It is based on the Taoist concept that everything is comprised of energy called Qi. When the energy in an environment is not flowing properly it can cause disharmony. Feng Shui works to balance this energy in order to achieve greater productivity, happiness, and health.

The Lo Pan varies from the simple Eight Directions to elaborate instruments which include the full 360 degrees of a circle, and twenty-four directions known as the Twenty-Four Mountains, and various intricate formulas relating to the directions. This allows the practitioner to be extremely detailed when they make a Feng Shui determination.

Like Qigong and Tai Chi Chuan, Feng-Shui is a study and practice of how energy moves and how to direct it. There are several different schools of Feng Shui. The most common Form School method considers Qi flow in and around objects and land formations to find the most auspicious flow of energy to align homes, gardens, businesses, and grave sites.

For instance, in a house the map would be oriented to the front door. Each of the nine areas on the Feng Shui map corresponds to a quality like relationships, wealth, health etc. The objects in each of these areas are positioned to encourage an auspicious flow of energy. Certain colors, plants, chimes, mirrors, and other remedies are used to improve a particular situation. Feng Shui recognizes that all living and non-living things are connected. If one thing is out of place it can affect other areas of our life.

In Feng Shui maps, the center of the Ba Gua is represented by the Earth element. The Earth element is seen as fundamental and the source of all other elements. In the peasant home, the kitchen stove is usually in the center. The stove was central because it was used for cooking and providing heat. The center of the Feng Shui map represented Health. Our ability to perform any activity is determined by our health.

Magic Square

Feng Shui means "wind-water." Feng-Shui is used to keep evil spirits away and increase good Qi. It uses what is called the Magic Square, based on the Later Heaven Model of the Ba Gua to illustrate this movement.

The Magic Square is divided into nine parts in a square of three by three. The order has a specific arrangement where the numbers of any line of three add up to fifteen. The numbering system creates a path of Qi which is powerful and considered magical.

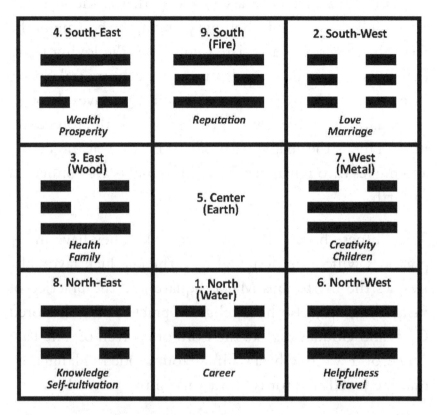

Image of The Magic Square Janet Seaforth collection.

If we consider the Three Powers and the Three Treasures on this configuration, the top three squares represent Heaven, the middle three represent humanity and the bottom three represent Earth. Heaven has come down to the plane of earth in the northwest which signifies travel and helpful people. The Earth is in the heavenly plane in the Southwest which is the square of marriage. It reminds me of the old quote, "Marriages may be made in heaven, but they have to be lived on earth."

If we impose a human figure on the Square their head would be in Fire and their feet in Water. Water sinks and fire rises. Jing energy is associated with the kidneys and water. It begins at the Bubbling Spring in the bottom of the feet. Shen energy is associated with fire, the loving light, that lives in our heart and mind as the Immortal Spirit. Fire from our heart rises to our mind. Qi moves through the squares from the bottom center one, to the top center nine. This is the magic path of Qi. Earth is at the center and moves through all levels, as all elements are connected to earth.

The Chinese have a deep belief in luck. They have many practices which are designed to influence luck favorably. Besides the mysterious Magic Square and the practice of Feng Shui, they also have religious practices that honored Gods and Goddesses, like the Lord of Heaven or The Jade Emperor. I was told by a Chinese tour guide in Hangchow that the Jade Emperor is known in China as Mr. Heaven.

The Jade Emperor and the Kitchen God

I learned about the Jade Emperor when I stayed at the Dragon Tiger Temple, which was also Sifu's house. I'd watch Sifu float around the kitchen as he gracefully prepared his herbal concoctions, lifting the drape of his robe as he reached his long, dark arm across the counter to choose a bit of herb. He moved slowly, evenly, calmly, like he was doing Tai Chi. While he was doing this, he'd carry on a delightful conversation, often chuckling as he told his stories. The beauty of his movements filled me with joy. I wanted my everyday movements to flow like Tai Chi.

I noticed how he kept his kitchen as well. The house was a two-story Salt-Box style early American country home, with the kitchen in the back. He had a kitchen garden just out the back door that he used in his medicinal cooking. The house reminded me of an old Southern mansion with its four big pillars holding up a veranda. The front porch stretched the entire length of the house with a full balcony above. The east side of the house looked out on the rising sun over the Sonoma Valley of the Moon. It was perfect that this holy man would take up lodging there and eventually make it into a Taoist Temple. He had it consecrated by a Taoist priest from San Francisco as Lung Lu Shan Tzu or Dragon Tiger Mountain Temple. This was the birthplace of my Tai Chi practice and the site of my Taoist consecration on June 21st Father's Day, 1978, year of the Earth Horse.

As I sat up on the end of the counter watching Sifu flip the ingredients of veggies and herbs in his wok, I noticed a funny little paper taped up on the back of the stove. "What's that?" I asked him. He informed me that the peasants of China hang a paper "Kitchen God" at the back of the stove to ensure good health and abundant harvest. A few days before the new year the paper is burned, after smearing its mouth with honey. This releases the God back to heaven. The honey ensures that the Kitchen God will give a good report to the Jade Emperor in Heaven of how the family is doing. After thoroughly cleaning the kitchen, a new kitchen God is installed as part of the New Year's celebration. The duty of hanging the kitchen god is performed by the man of the house.

The poor peasants of China worked hard to feed their family. The stove was the center of the house and nourishment. This simple paper Kitchen God gave them hope against famine and encouragement to be kind to one another as the Jade Emperor in Heaven was watching. The husband's duty of hanging a new Kitchen God brought his attention to answering to Heaven for cultivating his crops and maintaining the health of his family.

Chinese Martial Arts

Shaolin

There are Five Sacred Mountains in China. The central and highest is Songshan in the Shaoshi or Song mountain range, in Henan province. It is home to the Shaolin Temple. Shaolin means Monastery in the forest or woods of Shaoshi Mt. It was founded in 495 CE by an Indian monk, named Batuo. He gained favor with emperor Wu and was given this site. The Shaolin Temple is renowned as the birthplace of the Chinese martial arts. Batuo means "man with consciousness."

Emperor Wu granted the temple as a place where the monks could transcribe Sanskrit texts into Chinese script so that

Chinese Buddhists could have a better understanding of the Buddhist religion.

The Shaolin Temple burned down several times through the ages and was rebuilt. The last time was during the Cultural Revolution when many books and records of techniques were destroyed. Martial artists make pilgrimages to the site for training. I went to the Wushu Championships in China with Sifu Justin Eggert, who spent many months training there.

Bodhidharma

A Buddhist monk from India named Bodhidharma, or Daruma, came to the palace of Emperor Wu and assisted him with the translations of the Buddhist Sanskrit. Bodhidharma told Emperor Wu that he gained no merit in granting the Shaolin temple. It was only by his own internal process of mind that he would reach Nirvana, not by good deeds. Bodhidharma left the palace and made his way to the Young Forest monastery. Legend says the monks refused to let him in. Maybe he was too strange. So, he went to a cave nearby and sat in meditation. It is said he sat for nine years. By that time, the monks were begging him to come out and teach them. A classic story tells of one monk that cut off his hand to get Bodhidharma's attention, and eventually Bodhidharma relented. He began teaching. He saw the monks were out of shape from long hours bent over translating the Sanskrit and sitting in meditation.

Buddhists are not aggressive. They don't start fights, but they need to defend themselves. Perhaps Bodhidharma learned to fight as he traveled the Silk Road and other paths that were known to be dangerous due to gangs of bandits. He designed a series of exercises known as The Eighteen Hands of Bodhidharma that loosen the joints and have martial applications.

I was introduced to Bodhidharma by my sister Caron. I visited her in the 60's in Mill Valley north of the Golden Gate. Caron was beautiful, enchanting, and fun. I was a young teen and dazzled by her bohemian, beatnik charm. She put a small well carved ceramic netsuke of Bodhidharma in my palm and said it would bring me luck. He was an ugly man with a bug-eyed face. His upturned head rested in one hand. A leg and foot came out of his round belly which had a crescent moon on it. The bottom of the netsuke displayed a Chinese chop mark. Caron told me to put it on my window sill during any eclipse. It was a duty I took seriously.

I was told Bodhidharma had only one arm and one leg. Because he meditated so deeply, he was slowly disappearing back to heaven. He was the father of Zen or Chan Buddhism.

Chang San Feng and Wu Dang

Some scholars believe Chang San Feng was a legendary figure, but I was taught and believe that Chang San Feng was a real person. He is considered the founder of Tai

Chi Chuan. Chang was in a class of scholar warriors or "shi" and knew the classics. The emperor wanted him to serve in his court, but Chang preferred to be a hermit. He escaped to Wu Dang Mountain. This is one of the Five Sacred Mountains and part of a small mountain range in Hubei Province in northwestern China. Known for its Taoist temples, Wu Dang became the counterpart to Shaolin Temple, and was renowned for the practice of Tai Chi Chuan.

Born on April 9th, 1247 CE, Chang San Feng's legend says he lived over 200 years. Chinese legends contain many stories of hermits, martial artists, monks and Taoists who lived extraordinarily long lives. Chang San Feng was described as a Hsien or Xian, a Taoist term for an inspired sage, a person with superpowers, a magician.

In the late 13th century Chang stayed at the Shaolin Temple. Some of the monks had become unhealthy and weak from long hours of translating texts and sitting in meditation. Those that practiced martial arts had degenerated, losing their compassionate spirit, and relying on muscle strength and brute force. Chang wanted to bring martial arts practice into alignment with Taoist principles.

The symbol of the Snake and the Crane is an icon in martial arts. Sifu told me Chang San Feng prayed and meditated out of his concern for the monks. He looked out his window wondering how he could help them and happened to see a fight between a snake and a crane. The crane swooped in with its big wings spread to attack the snake. The snake twisted and turned away from the strike. The crane attacked again. The snake recoiled and struck back. The crane lifted its leg to avoid the bite. They fought until they were both exhausted. The snake slithered off, and the crane flew away.

Chang realized that he had been witnessing a perfect exhibition of the I Ching principles of adapting to change and blending soft and hard, strength and yielding. The continuity and flow of the circular movements seemed in accord with his Taoist observations of nature.

This story is incorporated in the Tai Chi movements of Crane Spreads its Wings and Snake Creeps Down. The snake is yin Earth. It lies close to the ground. It is a symbol of healing and herbal medicine. Seen in the depiction of Nu Wa and Fuxi whose lower bodies are entwined in the forms of two snakes, it represents the roots of our existence. The crane is yang Heaven. It is seen as symbolizing longevity, immortality, happiness, and good fortune. It is the messenger of the Gods and intermediary between Heaven and Earth. It represents higher states of consciousness and the ability to travel to other worlds. Pictures of cranes are often placed in coffins.

Chang San Feng restored grace and philosophy to the Taoist martial arts when he designed a martial form, called Tai Chi Chuan, which incorporated the concepts of Taoism, I Ching, Five Elements, Eight Directions and Yin/Yang theory.

Ba Gua and Tai Chi Chuan

In Tai Chi practice we use the Before Heaven model of Ba Gua. Our practice is enriched by knowing the directions and their correspondences to the I Ching. We also become familiar with how each direction represents a position in the Confucian family.

In the form, we begin with Wuji and connect with the vertical directions of Heaven above, Earth below, and our Humanity between them. Then our focus moves to the horizontal directions which anchor the movements. In the Dragon Tiger Mountain Tai Chi form, the practitioner begins facing north, the direction of Earth and the Great Unknown from which creation emerges in the form of yin and yang. The north is represented in the Confucian family as the Mother. After paying our respects with the Kuan Li bow, we take a conscious breath. Our hands are alert at our sides, as we connect and sink into the energy of solid mother earth. We fill with Qi as we inhale and our arms float up towards heaven, the light, the majesty of the cosmos. This is a return to noticing our posture in vertical alignment.

The Ba Gua is the heart of Taoist philosophy and the pattern for Tai Chi forms. Movements of the form take us through the many phases of the Ba Gua. With the first movement we turn to the west, the direction of the moon and Water. We continue around the circle to the south which is Father Sky and Heaven. From the position of Universal Post, we reach out in Fan Woman to the southeast, Joyous Lake and the youngest daughter. The movement Sparrow Spreads its Wings carries us to the opposite direction in the northwest, the Mountain, and the youngest son.

The individual movements also reflect nature. As we become the Crane Standing on One Leg, we feel the power of Grasping the Sparrows Tail, and the humility of Embracing the Tiger. I am intrigued by the poetry of the names such as "Clouds Touch the Mountain Tops," "Fair Woman Works the Shuttle," "Repulse the Monkey." My mind is full of images as I move my center of gravity, filling and emptying my weight in rhythm with my breath. I extend and recoil. I float through the movements, expanding and gathering Qi.

A martial arts practitioner can choose how to respond to an opponent. She can disappear like fog, resist like a mountain, or fight back like a tiger.

Chinese Internal Martial Arts

Tai Chi Chuan, Hsing-I, and Ba Gua

Chinese martial arts are now called Wushu, which means martial arts, and are considered a sport. Before the Cultural Revolution they were called Kung Fu or Gong fu, which means work accomplished. Gong, work, is like the gong in Qigong, and fu means penetrating heaven. There are three major internal styles of Kung Fu. They are Tai Chi Chuan or Taijiquan, Hsing-i Chuan, and Ba Gua Zhang. Ba Gua is practiced walking in a circle. Hsing-i is practiced in straight lines. Tai Chi is oriented to the Eight Directions as a square within a circle and invokes spiral energy.

Hsing-i or Xing Yi Quan means Form-Intention Fist or Shape-Will Fist. It refers to the ability of the mind to create an idea and project it into the body. It is considered the most yang of the internal arts. Hsing-i uses intention of the mind to direct the form. The practitioners of Hsing-i are militant, marching in straight lines, with a powerful emphasis at the end of every technique on mentally and physically taking an enemy down. Punching and striking movements are done in straight lines, at normal speed with explosive power. Hsing-i never retreats. As an internal martial art, rather than using muscular tension for power, Hsing-i emphasizes relaxation, intentional Qi, and stillness of mind.

My Tai Chi sister Michelle Dwyer practiced Hsing-i. She said it was created by a guy in prison whose cell was long and narrow, therefore the forms are short and straight. During some of our Spring Trainings she taught several of the forms. They were physically demanding requiring strength, stamina, and flexibility.

Like Tai Chi, Ba Gua Zhang also applies the philosophy of the Eight Directions, the basis of the I Ching. Its name means Eight Trigram Palm. Sifu Nam Singh said that Ba Gua Zhang is the deadliest practice in the Chinese martial arts.

Although Ba Gua Zhang originated with the "mountain people," it was designed as a close-quarter combat art. The use of a circular form requires the student to master subtle curvature change while in motion. The student integrates curves and angles into the depth of the sinews and joints and is able to maneuver to easily overtake and neutralize an opponent.

I've had the privilege to study Ba Gua Zhang from several practitioners. My first experience was with a teacher who visited Sifu in Sonoma. It was fascinating to feel the smooth circular patterns which can change abruptly with foot work and the maneuvering of the arms and palms. I tried to keep up but felt very awkward and he wasn't interested in working with women. The next few Ba Gua classes were at PAWMA camp with several Chinese masters.

At one of the camps, I trained with a woman from the east coast. She had been totally committed, for about ten years, to Ba Gua Zhang practice. In Ba Gua Zhang practice, you can walk alone or in a group. Our group of about sixty women practiced circle walking in an open area in the woods. She had us slide into our steps as if rolling a little stick under our feet. Then she had us take a firm empty step as if we were holding down the head of a snake. Our arms were held outstretched in various shapes which cultivated qi. We walked for about an hour. It was exhausting but exhilarating.

The arms and hands have specific postures to increase Qi power, muscle strength, and to promote healing. The palm positions are exact. The Lotus Palm practice enables each finger to be a flexible potent weapon while simultaneously being trained as a healing instrument. Each finger is stretched and reaches out forming a whole in the same way that petals of a flower form a whole. The eyes are concentrated as if aiming the energy emitted from the fingers.

Ba Gua is also practiced by partners in application drills, like Tai Chi Chuan's partner work, which is called Push Hands. The routines teach neutralizing a strike by employing subtle pressures and leverages to subdue an opponent. Using the slightest touch, one can redirect and turn an opponent's energy. This is the principle of moving a thousand pounds with four ounces of force.

Push Hands

Push Hands practice intrigues me, and I had an aversion to it. The first time Sifu Nam Singh worked with me, we faced each other with the back of our wrists touching. The soft interchange of energy was so intense I started to cry.

Push Hands practice teaches us to maintain the round shape of our arms and to expand and extend Qi in what is called peng force. Push hands practice makes our Tai Chi form powerful.

Sifu Nam Singh would have us partner with another student about our same size. We faced each other and began with the posture of Universal Post, as if we were holding a big bubble with our arms to establish our own energy field. Then we took a right bow stance with the forward foot in alignment with and inside our partner's forward foot. The back of our right wrists touched lightly, like two wings on a butterfly. Push Hands teaches sensitivity to our own energy and to another energy field. The partners are always physically connected. This connection is called "sticky hands."

As one partner moves forward in a push, the other receives the push and turns at the waist to deflect the force. When the force is deflected, the roles are reversed. Partner B now pushes towards partner A, and A turns in deflection. Push Hands is a continuous play of sending and receiving energy. Each player has their own bubble of Qi which adheres to the other player's bubble of Qi. It is a sensitivity exercise of sending, receiving, and redirecting energy.

Yang energy moves in a positive direction. It is expanding energy. The yin energy is still or retreating in a negative direction. Yin is condensing energy. A step forward contains the intention to withdraw; a step backwards always includes the intention to advance. Tai Chi movements are done with relaxation. The appearance is soft like cotton while the inside is strong like steel. This level of achievement is called "needle inside cotton." Yin/yang are in balance. Being strong inside and soft outside gives you yang in yin, and yin in yang. When we are still and grounded, the expansive or explosive moving yang energy can be more powerful because it has a solid yin base.

Push Hands taught me to integrate my whole body. I couldn't move anyone with just my arm. The strength of force came from my ability to ground, to come from my center line of gravity, to gather power from my lower dan tien and project with my whole body into the center of my partner.

There are many Push Hands forms, some using both arms to manipulate the energy flow. It can take years to master the skill. Masters are incredibly soft, detecting the point of balance in their partner and uprooting them with effortless skill.

The Push Hands competitions I have seen were disappointing. I thought they looked like Sumo wrestlers. This was not moving 1000 pounds with 4 ounces of energy as in the Tai Chi way. But when I worked with heavy-weight champion Stephen Watson, I felt an energy field that enveloped both of us. As I pushed towards his center he quickly and gently redirected my force aside. It was like there was nothing there to push against and I was put off balance. To maintain my balance, I learned to sink my center in spiral force. My recoil could be used to find his center's edge and change his direction.

Michelle Dwyer taught Push Hands at my school's Spring Trainings. She used many methods and forms, but my favorite was Da Lu. Da Lu uses the trigrams of the I Ching and Ba Gua. In the Push Hands practice of Da Lu, the outside shape of the Four Corners is represented by a circle and their inside shape is a square. The cardinal points North, South, East and West are seen as an inner circle and represent Heaven. The corners provide the square representing Earth. Each direction is assigned a partner movement and a self-defense application.

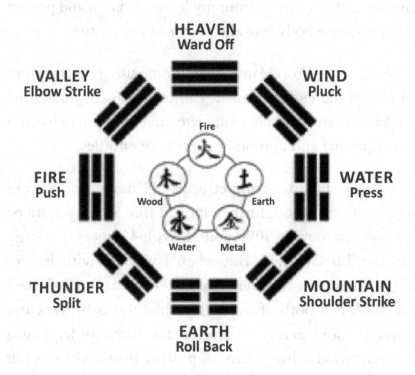

Peng, ward-off, is an expansive bubble-like energy represented by Chien, heaven, in the South.

Lu, roll-back, is a receptive energy, which can control a thousand pounds with four ounces of force by redirecting it. It is represented by Kun, earth, in the North.

Chi, press, is sticking to an opponent with a hand, arm, shoulder or back like water drilling into a crack. It is represented by Kan, water, in the West.

An, push, is feeling the opponent's strength and yielding until the right moment comes to apply force. It is represented by Li, fire, in the East.

Tsai, pull-down, is unbalancing an opponent by using your whole body to pull down on an opponent's arm. It is represented by Sun, the Chinese word for wind, in the Southwest.

Lieh, split, is grasping and twisting an opponent's wrist, then stepping behind an opponent to trip them, strike, or push their chest. It is represented by Chen, thunder, in the Northeast.

Chou, elbow-strike, is a surprise strike with the elbow. It is represented by Tui, lake, in the Southeast

Kao, shoulder-strike, is a close-in strike using the shoulder, pelvis, and hip in unison. It is represented by Ken, mountain, in the Northwest.

Weapons

Tai Chi Chuan has many forms that utilize various weapons. I've practiced several including staff, spear, sword, and fan. The fan is a subtle weapon which could have metal ribs like knives with sharp ends that slice or stab an opponent. Staff and sword practice loosens and strengthens the wrists, arms, shoulders and body core.

Sifu said "It takes one hundred days to learn staff, and one thousand days to learn sword." Both the staff and the sword are extensions of the body. Our inner Qi is projected out into the staff, or the cutting edge or point of the sword. When we practice with weapons, we extend our Qi Field.

The same principles of Tai Chi apply to weapons practice. The Essential Qualities of Evenness, Slowness, Clarity, Balance and Calmness come into play. Practicing slowly and evenly creates clarity and accuracy when the forms are executed quickly. In general, all movements in weapons forms are aligned to the Eight Directions. Your field of operation in Tai Chi is as large as your "reach." When working with a weapon, it extends to the tip of your weapon. You can feel the power of the circle as the staff or sword whips around gathering energy for a strike. Your Qi is extended through your weapon in strikes, jabs, and stabs. The yin circle gathers the power for a yang strike.

The Staff

Sifu took some of his students to Chinatown in San Francisco to pick out staves. The staves had to be straight and approximately one hand higher than our head. We'd measure the correct height with our fingers stretched out, our thumb on top of our head and our little finger reaching up. The cheapest were bamboo. They usually had rubber tips on the ends and the bamboo could take quite a beating.

Partner practice with staves is downright fun. Your speed and accuracy are tested. The rewards and defeats are instant. I quickly learned to be more aware of how to protect my body from an oncoming blow and immediately offer a counter attack. When we drilled, the staves struck against each other, making loud hollow sounds, which added to the excitement.

The Sword

Sifu Nam Singh taught the classic Tai Chi Chuan weapons of staff and sword. He instructed us to bring the Chinese classic double-edged sword and the saber to class if we wanted to learn Tai Chi sword forms. Of course, I wanted to learn these ancient arts, but I didn't have the money or way to order the prescribed weapons. So, I went to the Army Surplus store to see if they had any swords. They did. I found a nice machete for five dollars. When I took it to class, Sifu laughed and then looked horrified. He said no one was allowed to use a "live" blade in class. I told him I would be very careful, but he said absolutely not! He generously gave me his wooden sword, made of rosewood, which I still treasure and use.

The metal sword is a mystical instrument. Of the Three Treasures, Qi is Air, Jing is water, and Shen is fire. Air is associated with the element of metal, the mind and the upper dan tien. The mind is described as having characteristics like a sword. A discerning mind cuts through to reveal the truth.

The sword is compared to the brush of Chinese painting and calligraphy. Like the brush it must be imbued with

Qi. Both the brush and the sword should be handled with spontaneity.

Learning to work with weapons requires a higher level of commitment. You must be respectful of their added power. When we bow with a weapon, our right hand comes to our heart. The fingers are upright, pointing to heaven to signify an extra measure of compassion.

Punch

When throwing a punch, we move from our core out. The final turn of the wrist comes from the grounding of the feet and the strength in the legs. Manifestation of energy comes up through the lower dan tien to the chest, shoulder, elbow and is finally expressed through the wrist and hand. The fist in a punch is much more effective if it comes from this spiral energy. As the fist connects with its target, it spirals like a screw to move energy deep into the opponent.

Spiral Power

The spiral is the powerful form of energy that shapes hurricanes, our solar system, our Milky Way galaxy, and the code of our inheritance, the DNA molecule.

Sifu said that when we stand in meditation, we can think of ourselves in the calm eye of the hurricane. Chaos may surround us, but we can keep our focus on the still center. Likewise, as we move in Tai Chi forms, the center of calm moves with us. We direct and redirect the energy in expanding spirals or gather in our energy with coiling power.

Sifu had a symbol for spiral power in the form of a dorje on his altar. The dorje is a double-sided instrument capped on each side by four prongs coming together at the polar ends. It depicts energy changing form and represents a thunderbolt. The shape of the dorje forms an infinity sign, a spiral of yin and yang in all directions. The dorje is a symbol held by Kuan Yin to show She has the power of all possible possibilities.

Tai Chi movements are based on spiral power. By emphasizing the spiral nature of the movement, we gain more force. The energy comes up through the earth, is manifested in the lower dan tien and waist and has its final expression in the hands. Think of a snake coiling to make use of its power to strike. We can spiral out to express energy and we can spiral in to gain power. We use the spiral to direct and redirect energy.

> # We spiral out to express energy. We spiral in to gain power.

Most people in the beginning of their Tai Chi practice overextend. They throw their arms around outside their field of influence. The power of Tai Chi come from the axis. The arms stay in a wide angle in front of the body. Most movements stem from the posture of Universal Post. It establishes our reach. Beyond our reach we have little influence.

Practice Fourteen:
Carry the Ball of Qi

Use spiral energy to work your core around
your axis and pump your lymph.

Your feet are positioned in a horse stance, parallel and
more than shoulder width apart. Your forearms are level
at your chest and your elbows are held slightly in from the
Universal Post position. The Qi Ball is held between your
palms. Sink down, by bending your knees and lower the
Qi ball to the Sea of Qi (lower dan tien). Your shoulders
stay relaxed.

Shift your weight to your right foot, remaining upright
without leaning. Turn your body, spinning around your
axis to the left. The ball stays in front of the lower dan tien
and now faces at a diagonal to the left. With the exhale,
push off with the right foot, shifting your weight to your
left foot. Now the ball is facing the outside of the body.
With an inhale, turn on your axis, turning the waist to
the right. Exhale and carry the Qi ball towards the empty
right foot. Feel the right foot fill as you gradually put your
weight on it. Keep the Qi ball in front of the lower dan
tien. When the right foot is full, or weighted, inhale as
you spin left. Turn on your axis, working your core. Push
off from the weighted right foot, and exhale as you move,
slowly and evenly to the left. When the left foot is full,
inhale while you spin to the right. Repeat by pushing off
with the left foot. Carry the weight of your body in your

hips and centered around your axis and relaxed. Move to the right, while carrying the Qi ball in front of your lower dan tien.

The gwa is the area in the crease of the leg at your hip where many lymph nodes reside. This area is pumped as you open and close the gwa. The gwa squeezes together as you move into your solid foot, and it opens as you unwind and spin. Inhale, spin, open the gwa. Moving into your solid foot, closes the gwa. Feel the pumping action as you cleanse your lymph glands and push the lymph through the body. Opening and closing the gwa is helpful in strengthening the immune system. You can feel one gwa close or squish, as your other gwa stretches and opens.

Reverse: Carry Qi ball with your weight on your left foot, turn around axis to left bringing the Qi ball to the outside of the body. Exhale as you **move backwards** to fill your right foot. The Qi ball is held directly in front of the lower dan tien. Inhale as you spin to face the outside turning right. Exhale, sit back as you move your weight on your left foot. Continue the pattern until you feel refreshed.

Spiral energy moves up from earth to foot to ankle to knee, hip, waist, and down from the dan tien which activates the movements. Arms and hands are stable and stay in front of lower dan tien, the Sea of Qi.

Spiral energy moves up and down in the direction we choose. We move from our feet up or from our head down. This spiral energy is important in Tai Chi. As directions change, the energy remains at the lower dan tien. Keep your shoulders level and avoid bouncing up and down. Energy is contained at the Sea of Qi.

Return to Center

Qigong and Tai Chi start and end with Simple Standing or Wuji. Often forms require returning to exactly where one starts. Here is a practice. Put a marker on the floor between your feet when you begin your form and see if you can return to the same mark. When you return to the same place, notice the difference in how you felt before your practice, and how you feel after completion. Do you feel more alive, connected, and peaceful? If you do, you know you had a good session.

NINE

Returning

Tai Chi and the Tao Te Ching

My beloved teacher Sifu Nam Singh told his students to read the <u>Tao Te Ching,</u> which means The Way and its Power. He said it would help us to understand the roots of Tai Chi Chuan. At first, I couldn't relate to very much of it, but I liked the way it started. It was simple and it included a feminine presence.

> *The Tao that can be named is not the everlasting Name.*
> *That which has no name is the origin of heaven and earth;*
> *That which has a name is the Mother of all things.*
> Chen man Ching translation

Reading these opening lines was my first experience with the Mother, as a revered presence. This was not in my Lutheran training. We worshipped God the Father, God the Son, and God the Holy Spirit. The Tao Te Ching honored nature and the feminine.

I found that when I did Qigong meditations or the Tai Chi form, I could feel the spirit that I had experienced in church. I went to church on Sundays with my mom, my brother Chuck, and my father, who came with us about once a month. We had a kind pastor. A feeling of peaceful joy came over me in prayer, in song, and sometimes during a sermon. I felt an uplifting as our spirits united. This feeling flooded our bodies and the room with lightness. The energy was far beyond dogma, guilt, or fear. It was atonement reached by blending our hearts and minds with the spirit of a loving God, touching into undeniable and boundless grace.

I became disillusioned with the church teachings at around fourteen years of age. I left the church because I found the regimented dogma was confining and alienated me as a woman. I also couldn't believe a merciful God would send people to hell if they didn't accept Jesus as their personal savior. I asked, "What about the people in Africa who have never heard of Jesus?" The pastor reassured me they would be judged on their own merits, but if they had the chance to accept Jesus and rejected him then they too would be dammed. I realized I never wanted to be a missionary as it could get people in everlasting trouble. I figured they were better off not knowing than to take a chance on a misunderstanding.

Even though I rejected the church, I've always considered myself a Christian. I felt I could be a Christian without church membership because I held on to the premise that

Jesus gave us, which is that God's law is "written in our heart and in our mind," Hebrews 10:16. In Qigong, I believe this is Shen, the Immortal Spirit, which is imbued with loving light that lives in our heart and mind.

I believe Jesus traveled the Silk Road to India and was introduced to Eastern thought and Buddhism. When he returned to the west, he gave a new commandment to love one another as God loves us. Mother told me Jesus invited humanity, as the church, to be the bride, the beloved, the feminine form of the masculine creative force. The bride is tender, mature, responsive, and cherished. Humanity takes its place in relationship to the creative loving light of heaven on earth. My mother was always a romantic. I guess I am too.

Referred to in the first chapter of the Tao Te Ching, I see "the Mother of all things" as the birth of material existence. From the birth of creation, it took billions of years before form took shape in our universe. On earth, Mother Nature consists of intricately interconnected forms that change constantly. We understand nature through observation, and we name the many forms that nature takes.

There is a chaotic thing, born before heaven and earth,
So silent, so empty, unique and unchanging, circling endlessly.
It could be considered the Mother of all under heaven.
I do not know its name.
I reluctantly style it "Tao"
And if forced to, reluctantly describe it as "great"
Chapter 25 Translation by Chen man Ching.

The power that brought the Cosmos into being from the initial point of singularity remains a mystery. It is that which has no name. It is beyond words. The author of the Tao Te Ching used the word "reluctantly" because he recognized the fallacy of using a name for the unnamable. I think this is similar to many religions that don't say the name of God or decline to depict it in art, like the Jews and the Muslims. It is too powerful, too great, to be defined by word or art.

The Tao gives birth to Tai Chi. It creates the yin and yang which are depicted as two fish swimming in the Tai Chi symbol. Basically, yang is cause or force and yin is the effect or form. The dance of yin and yang is produced from the unnamable Tao, constantly creating through change or movement.

Lao Tzu was advocating the very things Tai Chi promotes, which are the yin qualities of softness and stillness. The mysterious yin is dark, intuitive, fecund. We are instructed to be like a valley that holds all and receives the power of the creative yang.

The Valley Spirit never dies.
It is named Mysterious Female.
And the Doorway of the Mysterious Female
Is the base from which Heaven and Earth Spring.
Chapter 6, Tao Te Ching

In Qigong and Tai Chi, nature is celebrated and imitated with our body, mind, and spirit. We stand like a crane, spread our wings and rise like a phoenix, crouch down like a snake, our hands touch the mountain tops like clouds.

The Feminine

Tai Chi Chuan is based on the principles of the feminine. Other martial arts often require strength, but Tai Chi requires being soft, open, and paying attention to energy. We feel the movement in the stillness, the stillness in the movement. Tai Chi Chuan is a cooperative movement. We practice being in tune with others and moving in unison. These are feminine qualities that give strength and power to the creative masculine qualities within each person. The yin holds the yang like the earth holds the light of the sun. We receive the energy and are responsive to it. The balance of yin and yang are the heart of Tai Chi Chuan.

Lao Tzu Rides an Ox

The Way and its Power, the Tao Te Ching, was written 2500 years ago. It is the oldest book of Taoist philosophy. Its roots are obscure. Even Lao Tzu may be a compilation of several scholars who wrote down the Taoist knowledge which had previously been an oral tradition. Lao Tzu simply means "old man." The story goes, before Lao Tzu left on an ox to an unknown land, the gatekeeper at the mountain pass asked him to write down the wisdom of the Taoists.

I see the story of Lao Tzu leaving on an ox as operating on a symbolic level. Lao Tzu is passing through the gate from one world to another, from a time of matriarchy and oral tradition to the patriarchal time of the written word.

For me, the ox symbolizes the matriarchy from which the Taoist sensibilities emerged in the time of the Wu. The ox is a symbol of earth energy and femininity. Oxen helped people till the soil. It is a beast of burden, powerful, and subservient.

In Chinese astrology, the ox is the second animal of the twelve-year cycle. It is the yin aspect to the yang rat. In the story of the twelve animals of the calendar, the rat, in order to win the race, transverses the river riding on the ox's horns. Then scampering quickly to the Jade Emperor (Lord of Heaven), the rat was awarded with starting each new twelve-year cycle.

The Tao Te Ching was written down many centuries and dynasties after the time of the Wu. Confucius arrived on Lao Tzu's heels. Confucian doctrine became widespread over two thousand years ago. Slowly this patriarchal structure diminished the power of women. Women were dependent on the oldest son, who inherited the family home and business. Women were reduced by Confucian philosophy to be obedient to their husbands and to bear his children. Women's power, as shamen, went underground. The word Wu was degraded and translated as "witch."

Kuan Yin: Goddess of Fearless Compassion

In 1977, I was longing for a feminine voice in my spiritual practice. My Sifu introduced me to the Goddess of Fearless

Compassion known as Kuan Yin. I saw a white porcelain statue of Her, in his dining room, in a glass case with other figurines and fine vases. She was the depiction of a lovely lady in long robes with her head covered. She was serene, quiet, and had a quality of listening. She held a small vase in her hand. Sifu said it was her bottle of Sweet Dew which she used to cure all the ills of the world. The dew forms on the grass about four a.m. It is the best hour for meditation. It is quiet and dark. Perhaps all our woes can be healed by the act of meditation which gives us new perspective and insight.

Kuan Yin is commonly known as the Goddess of Mercy and "She who hears the cries of the world." She is the most beloved Goddess of the Chinese. She is considered Buddhist and a feminine form of the male god Avalokitesvara, "the lord who looks upon the world with compassion." I believe she was probably originally a fertility Goddess as she is also the "Giver of Children." She is associated with the Tibetan Goddess White Tara, also a Goddess of Compassion, though Kuan Yin is much more serene. Tara's depiction often has one bare breast, while Kuan Yin is fully clothed.

Buddhist Bodhisattvas and Taoist Temples

Kuan Yin is known as a bodhisattva. A bodhisattva is one who refuses, or delays, going to heaven until all suffering on earth has ended. This reminded me of Dr. Martin Luther King's phrase, "Nobody is free, until everybody is free."

My favorite title for Kuan Yin is "Goddess of Fearless Compassion." This is Her challenge to us: Can you be fearless in your compassion? This state of power is derived from understanding and insight that come through the practices of meditation and cultivation of a compassionate heart. With practice, our compassionate presence becomes so strong that even fear dissolves into understanding.

Sifu Nam Singh encouraged his students to meditate. Sometimes we would sit on the floor of the Temple Room in his house. The Temple had been consecrated by the Taoist priest from San Francisco. The altar had to have the traditional wooden fish-shaped drum and a brass bell in the shape of a bowl. Sifu Nam Singh would knock on the fish with a mallet to invoke the deities and ring the bell at the beginning and end of meditation. It is common to have Taoist and Buddhist statues on Chinese altars. A large statue of Kuan Yin stood with the Eight Immortals of Taoist lore who were represented by eight ceramic statues that took their place beside her. Other Taoist deities were there, but two of them, The Jade Emperor and Tin How Ma, had prominence. Tin How Ma is also known as Mazu, the Queen Mother of Heaven. It is common for Chinese temples to be both Taoist and Buddhist. The three main religions of China: Taoism, Buddhism, and Confucianism, are complementary not competitive.

Sifu took some of his students to the Tin How (Tienhau) Temple in San Francisco on Waverly Place in the middle of Chinatown. While we were there, he would stop at his favorite shops. He stood out as a tall, black man, wearing the silk suits of another era. Sifu was known in the shops that sold temple incense and other things used in Taoist worship. The shop keepers would say, "Ah, Nam Singh, how are you?" The owner would often take him aside and tell him about some new item he may like to purchase for his temple. Sifu had impeccable taste and, although he was not at all wealthy, he bought only the finest quality.

The Tin How Temple is easy to miss. It is just a doorway with a sign above it, founded in 1852. It is the oldest Taoist temple in the city. I believe the temple was first erected by the grateful sailors who crossed the Pacific Ocean to work in California during the Gold Rush. It has suffered earthquakes and disrepair but was reconsecrated in 1975. It now resides on the top of the building on the fourth floor. We had to go up many stairs to find this simple shrine. Exhausted by the climb, we entered breathless as we bowed to the old woman who greeted us in Chinese. Sifu spoke a little Mandarin and Cantonese and the old woman nodded to us and directed us to come in. Like the stairs, the floors of the several rooms were old wood. The main room was naturally lit by the windows to the east. The balcony looked out onto the new Transamerica Pyramid building, giving us a feeling of being between the ancient and modern worlds. The rooms were full of various old dusty altars topped with kindly and fierce gods perched on silk brocades. These were attended by a few old women. They allowed Sifu to light incense.

On another excursion to San Francisco, we went to a Chinese temple where they honored Kuan Yin. It was full of Chinese families gathered in a casual atmosphere. There was a long table in the middle of the room filled with Chinese potluck. An altar was set up against one wall, and on the other end of the room a TV was left on. We chanted to Kuan Yin as we marched around the table. Many people used prayer beads. The beads flew through their fingers as they chanted at such a speedy pace that I couldn't get all the words in, but I did my best.

Lighting incense shows veneration of ancestors and is used in Chinese celebrations. During Chinese New Year, family members gather in their home village and visit the graves of their clan. Another interesting celebration is Chong Yang. From 25 CE, it has been celebrated in early October. It falls on the 9th day of the 9th month. Nine is an odd number. Odd numbers are yang. Double yang is considered dangerous. Therefore, it is suggested that on this day, one should climb a high mountain, drink chrysanthemum tea to cleanse the body, air out the house and visit graves to respect the ancestors. This event seems a little superstitious; however, these celebrations help people remember their ancestors, to cleanse their body, and to soften their heart.

I felt great affinity for the Taoist love of nature and their respect for those who came before them. But I especially loved Kuan Yin and wanted to know more about this fearless woman, so my Sifu gave me a book by John Blofeld, Bodhisattva of Compassion.

Celebrating the Sacred Feminine

Kuan Yin's Birthday

According to John Blofeld, the Chinese celebrate Kuan Yin's birthday on July 19th. For me it was a nice complement and balance to Christmas. We celebrate the Western, masculine Jesus in the yin winter, and celebrate the Eastern, feminine Kuan Yin in the yang summer.

I decided to celebrate her birthday on my little farm and invited the students from my various classes, who were all women at that time. We met in the meadow surrounded by madrones, firs, and oaks. Women would place an amulet, stone, a prayer, or flower on Kuan Yin's altar. The altar was simply a big, beautiful scarf laid out where the grass was still a little green on the edge of the woods, just under the trees. Incense would be lit and carefully placed in a large ceramic bowl filled with sand to hold the stick upright for our prayers and devotion.

We formed a circle and warmed up with Qigong moves, followed by our Tai Chi form. Tai Chi is often used to prepare for meditation. To celebrate and understand Kuan Yin, we wandered to a place of our choice around the meadow and woods, then sat in silent meditation. We contemplated her grace and found ways we could emulate her in our own life by being merciful, fearless, and serene. After about half an hour, I'd sound the gong, and we would return to Simple Standing in a circle. We would walk around in the circle chanting the Kuan Yin chant 108 times. This is the number of beads (nine times twelve) on a string of prayer beads. This necklace is often called a mala.

Kuan Yin's chant

Namo, Tai Chi, Tai Pi
Kuan Shi Yin, Pusa.

Translation:
Namo means Hail to Thee,
Tai Chi means Great, Complete Harmonious Energy,
Tai Pi means Grace
Kuan Shih Yin Pusa means
Kuan Yin sees and hears
and has the potent, patient, power
to teach and save us.

After the chanting we'd return to silence and the final Water Blessing, which I learned from Sifu. A small branch of a willow would be placed in a nice glass vase and set on the alter. The willow is sacred to Kuan Yin because it bends. It is not stiff but flexible. The vase was filled with blessed fresh water from the flowing creek. I would take the branch out of the water and splash water on all the recipients. Everyone loved it and would hold out their hands to catch the water and put it on their faces, rubbing in the blessings. Finally, we would share a potluck picnic feast.

Woman's Clan Retreat

At one of my many Kuan Yin birthday parties, a woman named Nympha came to celebrate with us. She had an extensive herb shop in the village of Mendocino and was known for her knowledge of healing and ancient women's culture. She was a "straga," a healer-witch from Sicily.

In 1996 she created an annual women's retreat, The Woman's Clan Gathering, and asked me to come and teach Qigong and Tai Chi. The Gathering met annually for almost a decade at a retreat in Albion. The five acres of land had apple orchards, a large grassy meadow, organic gardens of vegetables and flowers and a few majestic redwoods. There was a vintage house, and in the meadow next to it was a new Japanese style meditation hall and dorm rooms. I met many wonderful, powerful women from all over the country, including my beloved Marylyn Motherbear Scott.

One of the workshops late in the evening at Woman's Clan Gathering was Motherbear's "Bardic Circle." Motherbear is a substantial woman of Celtic heritage. She was dressed in flowing layered attire and held a wand-staff topped with a powerful crystal. She sat smiling like a Buddha as she directed the women to be seated. The circle of cushions surrounded a temporary altar made from scarves laid on the floor. On the sea of scarves was a bouquet of fresh flowers, crystals, prayer beads, and other items women had brought to receive the sacred energy generated by the ritual. Motherbear asked us to speak to the roots of our spiritual experience. We told our stories and passed her bejeweled wand as our "talking stick." Whoever held the stick had the attention and ear of all those in the circle. We were not interrupted and there was no cross talk. She made everyone feel noticed, included, and cared for. She was the Motherbear of the Bear Clan.

Goddess Gather

Motherbear and I created The Goddess Gather as a festival for women to honor the Divine Feminine presence within each of us. For over ten years we embodied different manifestations of the Goddess. We explored and experienced these womanly energies through presentations in workshops and performances. The day's workshops began in the early morning with Qigong and Yoga practice. They ended late in the evening with rituals, dancing, and performances. We were immersed in Goddess energy for three days.

We celebrated the loving energy of the Goddess with the freshness of children. We dressed like goddesses and expressed our inner selves through art projects. We danced and we sang, "The earth is our mother, and we take care of Her," along with many other Goddess songs of peace, joy, and reverence.

In 1998 I started hosting Kuan Yin's birthday celebration at The Goddess Gather. On Saturday afternoon I set up an altar with statues of Kuan Yin, an incense pot, flowers, and the items for the water blessing. Some women would place their own Kuan Yin statues or remembrances on the altar to receive energy. We lit memorial incense in honor of those who had died and those newly born. We each rang the gong and expressed a desire or request. This would be followed by a standing meditation with mudras, like the Kuan Yin Hands of Peace meditation.

You can do this meditation on your own to bring peace to yourself and the world.

Practice Form Fifteen: Hands of Peace

From a Simple Standing position, raise your arm with a soft elbow, slightly bent to just above shoulder height. The palm is forward as if you were waving. The other arm is to the side by the hip. Both palms are held facing forward projecting peaceful energy. Hold for about thirty-two breaths or five minutes and switch arms and repeat. Peaceful energy is sent from the palms out into the world.

You can also read the following meditation as a personal practice to engender feelings of peace and compassion.

> *Today I will feel at Peace. Within me is imperturbable peace.*
>
> *This peace is the root of my spirituality.*
>
> *This peace frames and reflects my mind's view of the world.*
>
> *This peace enables me to fearlessly trust my intuition.*
>
> *This peace is pure tranquility.*
>
> *The spiritually centered me is strong, power filled, positive and alive.*
>
> *Love radiates from my core and shines upon all those I encounter.*

Today I will feel no turmoil, no conflict.

I will not feel responsible for the thoughts and feelings of others.

Centered and composed, I will be clear about my limits, and I will forgive.

Perfect peace releases all stress and allows me to serenely experience all that comes my way.

Another practice I shared at the Goddess Gather was Awaken the Lotus. I love this practice because of the images it employs and because it expresses the body's range of motion. I have offered this Qigong meditation at various events, including a bridal shower and private retreats, and often end my classes with it. It can be wonderful as a short personal form. If you have only ten minutes for practice, this form gives you "good juice."

Practice Form Sixteen: Awaken the Lotus

Preparation: Assume the Simple Standing posture with your hands over your lower dan tien, below your navel. Your feet stand on the earth. Your head touches the Sky. Be like a water lily with roots in the mud, stem swaying in the water, flower reaching up to sun. Feel your breath in stillness until you are ready to move.

Gather Qi from Earth and Heaven: Inhale as you gather Qi from the earth and bring your hands up with your arms extended out to your sides all the way up to heaven. Gather heavenly Qi over the top of your head. Exhale bringing your hands down palms facing your body receiving Qi all the way to your feet. Repeat three times.

Morning Arises: With your palms facing the earth, extend your arms out at your sides, with your knees bent, like an umpire in baseball who is declaring a player is safe. Inhale as you bring your arms up and in, your elbows are slightly bent and your fingers are pointing forward, until your palms face each other, a few inches apart, at your heart level. Exhale as you bring your arms up in a big y shape with the palms up to face the sky. Your arms are spread as you lean back and look at the sky. Inhale as you bring your palms back to your heart level and exhale as you bring your hands back to face the earth. This movement is like the shape of an hour glass in that the hands are held wide at the sky and earth and narrow at the heart position. Repeat three times. On the last round when you are bringing your arms down from the heart, the knees don't bend as much and the palms turn to face forward at your sides, close to your body.

Lotus Awakens: The back of the hands push back. Your arms are fully extended and circle behind your body and up over the top of your head. When your arms are up over the top of the head touch the backs of the hands together. Turn your wrists and bring the heel of your hands and your fingertips together forming a lotus bud or prayer hands. Bring the lotus bud down to your heart level with the inhale, keeping your elbows held up. Exhale. As you inhale again, drop your elbow and open the lotus by spreading your fingers out to breath in its healing essence. As you exhale return to prayer hands. Feel your deep heart energy.

Clouds Part: From the prayer hands position, point your fingertips forward and extend your arms out in front at the level of the solar plexus. Bend at your hips, keep your back straight, look forward, maybe to the others in the circle. Turn your wrists so the palms face up, as if offering a gift of Qi to all those around you, and smile. Turn your wrists until the backs of your hands touch then separate them as you circle your arms out to your sides as far as you can all the way behind your back as if you are parting clouds. Your palms face each other, your fingers pointing behind you, your scapula are squeezed together, and you are still bent at the hips.

The Sunlight Reveals the Jewel Within: With your arms behind your back, bend your knees a little more and scoop up earth Qi with your hands. Both arms swing forward feeling into the grounding quality of the earth and rise like the sun to above your head. Bring in heavenly Qi then turn your wrists so the back of your fingers touch. The fingertips point into your body's centerline, starting at the top of your head. Then bring your arms down the front of your body slowly, and feel the Qi jewels sparkling in all your energy centers from your head to your feet. You may imagine different colored jewels at each of your chakras or just honor with gratitude all the wonderful parts of your body that work to keep you healthy and strong.

The Dew Returns to the Sky Above: Bend your knees. Your palms scoop imaginary dew from the earth as you squat. Inhale bringing your hands with the dew up to your heart level. Turn your hands over, giving a little dew to your heart. Exhale as you return the dew to the sky above, your wrists rotate, and your palms face upward as you push your palms to the sky. Look at the back of your hands. Face forward and inhale as your arms circle out and extend to your sides, palms face the earth, a little lower than your shoulders at heart level. Exhale as you continue the circle and return your palms to the lower dan tien bringing in the loving light and healing you've received. Take a few breaths. Feel the Qi. Feel that you are integrated and refreshed.

The dew forms on the earth about four o'clock in the morning.
This is the special hour of meditation when all is quiet and still.
It is said that the dew has the potent power to heal.

Meditation

Moving Qi and Returning to Stillness

The Tao abides in emptiness.
The whole universe surrenders to a mind that is still.
Silence and emptiness stimulate imagination
and sharpen perception.
Only through exercise can Tao be apprehended and expressed.
From Chuang Tzu

Meditation gives us a place to be still. The most common form of meditation is sitting in a chair, or on a cushion with the legs crossed. Meditation can also be done standing, walking, or lying down.

Qigong and Tai Chi are thought of as meditation in motion. They are also recommended to prepare a person for other forms of meditation. Sifu Nam Singh instructed us to take up a practice of sitting about fifteen to thirty minutes every day after we did our Tai Chi form. He suggested that we sit and listen to our breath and enjoy the results.

Sonoma Zen

I wanted to learn more about meditation. I joined the renowned Sonoma Mountain Zen Center for their early morning meditation. It was only about an hour away, up a narrow road, through the lovely landscape of Sonoma Mountain. The journey was as peaceful as the meditation. A large old barn was transformed into a meditation hall. It had a new wood floor and the practitioners sat on their round cushions all in rows, many in their monk's robes.

There was a feeling of respect for the silence and any noise was an obvious intrusion you didn't want to make. I could hear the breath of the people surrounding me. We sat for about an hour with our legs crossed, our hands in zazen posture with thumbs lightly touching, left hand supporting the right. It was the same mudra that we held in the Dragon Tiger Mountain form of Tai Chi Meditation Stance. It is the posture I still use while doing seated meditation. It gives me the best concentration and relative comfort.

I went to a few dharma talks at the center. Vow 43 states that only men can get into heaven. I asked a revered visiting teacher what he thought I should do about it. He answered, "Don't step on the grass." I didn't go back.

I purchased one of the sturdy black cushions that were made at the center. It was called a zafu. I think it cost $20 at the time. I know I couldn't afford the matching mat that went with the cushion. I still use my zafu, more than forty years later.

Being Still and Doing Nothing and
The Discomfort of Being Still

I've practiced sitting meditation for many years. Being still and doing nothing seems easy. But when you settle down the first thing that comes up is discomfort. It can be quite challenging. It's not very comfortable staying still. Sometimes it was downright painful. After a while I realized the pains come and go. I could experience the pain without moving away from it. I kept my position and breathed into the pain. I relaxed more deeply, opening the flows to alleviate the discomfort. If my lower back ached, I would let my energy sink down so I could feel myself resting on the earth. I would move slightly making minor physical adjustments. Or I would just be with the discomfort without trying to escape it. The condition would eventually change, as all things do. Just being with what was happening, without trying to change it, was a great relief.

Posture is Enlightenment

At one of the PAWMA camps held in the Los Angeles area, my students and I were delighted to practice an introduction to Vipassana, or Insight Meditation, with Sensei Michele Benzamine Miki. Michele is half Japanese. She had an elegant grace as she walked through the wooded camp in her Aikido hakima, with a sword slung on her belt and her black hair pulled into a long braid that hung down her back. She taught Aikido, Iaido sword and offered a meditation class. She was a fifth-degree black-belt; small, but exceedingly powerful. She was also fun and had an intriguing sense of humor. During her workshop on meditation, she gave instruction on posture techniques for endurance and sitting comfortably. I asked her what I could do about the pain I was experiencing between my shoulder blades when I sat in meditation. She said to lift my heart by raising my chest slightly, as if a string was attached lifting my heart up towards heaven. It helped. She also told us, "Some Zen teachers of meditation say, 'Posture is enlightenment.'" I think it's true. When you are in alignment, you can be open to the loving light of spirit. Like Wuji posture, this position puts us in alignment with earth and heaven so the energy can move through us.

Taking Refuge with Women

One of my students picked up a flyer at PAWMA camp that said Sensei Michele Miki was going to Sacramento to teach classes. She mentioned this to me and we decided to ask if she would consider coming to Mendocino County to teach us more about meditation. I got up the nerve to call her, and surprisingly, she said, "Yes."

Michelle suggested that our White Cloud Women's Temple School form a meditation sangha. A sangha is a community of people that comes together to meditate. We take "refuge" in the sangha. A refuge is a place to be free of danger, pursuit, or trouble. Finding a safe space to relax into meditation in the company of like-minded people supports and deepens our training.

We met at Po Yun Nei Kuan, on the farm. A Gatha, a verse by her teacher Master Thich Nhat Hanh, to be recited in rhythm with our breath, was printed on our program.

> *Entering the meditation hall*
> *I see my true self.*
> *Once I am seated*
> *All confusion vanishes.*

Ten women sat in a circle on cushions or in chairs. We lit a candle in the center of the circle. Michele had us go around the circle with a check-in using just three words to describe our body, emotion, and mind; like, "alert, excited, scattered". She directed us to take a comfortable posture and introduced us to the practice of "stopping to focus." She said we could use a candle, a mantra, or our breath. Then we moved into "Vipassana," looking deeply into the nature of what we are experiencing. We focused on the breath and allowed the awareness of other mind and body phenomena. After about thirty minutes, Michele had us do a standing meditation. She instructed us to take a powerful position, not passive or waiting. She told us to be deeply rooted in the earth like a tree. We held our arms like branches reaching to the sky and bearing the fruit of our insight. As we were visited by thought, sensations and emotions, she told us to remain still and accepting. Then we went outside and did a walking meditation. When she rang a big bell, we came back to the Tai Chi hall. The last position she taught was lying down on our backs. She said this was considered an advanced posture because it was difficult not to go to sleep in this position. I relaxed every place my body contacted the earth. The loving light of heaven felt like a sweet, soft blanket.

Michelle came up to teach many times in the 90's. After our first sessions I introduced her to my friend and colleague Sensei Gayle Fillman. Gayle was a high-ranking Aikido teacher who lived in Ukiah about an hour away. She was a big, blonde lesbian with a ready laugh. Her dojo was comprised of mostly agile men whom she threw around like tumble weeds. Gayle also worked with at-risk youth to restore their self-confidence. She used Aikido techniques in teaching gymnastics, taking her team to the California State Finals several times. Gayle and Michele formed a lasting friendship. We had several weekend Vipassana Meditation retreats for women, from our combined schools, in the mountains on Gayle's beautiful horse ranch.

We women strengthened our bodies with Qigong and Aikido warm-ups and softened our hearts with the formal practice of meditation. In the afternoon, after some free time, women would have a private audience with Michele. During the private sessions, in order to continue our mindfulness practice and get some exercise outside, I offered Tai Chi to the rest of the group as a moving meditation. We did the form in a meadow looking out at the tree lined, green fields of the Big Valley of Ukiah. The feeling of deep contentment and gratitude is an enduring memory, reminding me "the valley spirit never dies."

The Practice of Being Present

In Wuji we take time to be present. It is a form of meditation. We tune in to the stillness, to the emptiness and freshness of doing nothing. Standing meditation is the root of Qigong and Tai Chi. Most Qigong and Tai Chi forms begin with Wuji because all creative manifestations begin with the void. As we stand quietly in Wuji or move slowly in Tai Chi, we are aware of our breath. This awareness calms and centers us so we can let go of the endless stories of our mind, our illusions, and delusions. When we find ourselves lost in thought, we practice returning our attention to our breath. We connect to our heart's wisdom, the shen of our Immortal Spirit in the eternal present. We are relaxed but alert, the state of the warrior, the artist, the place of creative evolution.

> **Most Qigong and Tai Chi forms begin with Wuji because all creative manifestations begin with the void.**

Return to Presence

The future is a mystery.
The past is history.
Now is the gift.
That's why it's called the present.
From a favorite refrigerator magnet

When our mind is still and focused on our breath, thoughts naturally arise all the time. When we meditate, we let our thoughts float through without attachment or aversion. The thoughts are like clouds in a blue sky. We don't hold on to them. We neither cling nor avoid. We don't obsess. We simply bring the mind back to the breath in awareness. We just notice what is going on without trying to change it. Withdrawing from outer noise and chaos to the inner stillness of Wuji allows an awareness of loving light. When we turn our attention to receive it, it is always available. This is a place of peace. I call it "being open to the eternal present."

The eternal present gives me a sense of space in the moment. I can feel the expansiveness of not holding on to the past or future. When I am in the moment of now, I am free from thought of what I "should' have done or what I "have to" do. I can feel the edges of my constricted thinking expand as I breathe into tight places of guilt or shame or depression. The opportunity to see things differently arises in the space that is created by loosening my grip and letting go of my idea that I have to be a certain way to be acceptable as a person. In stillness I can see more clearly the way things are instead of dwelling on how I want things to be. I find that stillness cultivates a greater trust to let things unfold naturally. I am reminded by the sanity of stillness that I can only fix myself; I can't fix anyone else. We are unique and yet connected.

We are all alive through the elements of the Mother Earth and the spirit of Father Sky. Through our very breath, we take our place in the cradle of their love. We see the connection with all life on earth.

Path of Qi in the Micro-Cosmic Orbit

Sifu Nam Singh taught one of the most powerful practices I know. He taught us a Chinese breathing technique he called the Circulation of Light, which can be used to prepare for deeper meditation, increase energy, and connect the three dan tiens. This practice is also known as Micro-Cosmic orbit.

When I feel scared, frazzled, or have scattered energy, the Circulation of Light helps me center and settle down. I use it when I am stressed and tense, like when I am at the dentist. It helps me relax. I also use it when I am tired and slumping. It helps me straighten up, align my spine, and gives my organs more room so they can function properly. It is primarily used to cultivate Qi in the lower dan tien.

The Micro-Cosmic orbit is a profound breathing exercise. This stillness practice moves the Qi up your back through the Governing Channel, the major yang meridian, and down the front of your body, the Conceptual Channel, the major yin meridian.

> # The mind moves the Qi through the body, with the breath, and aligns the body between heaven and earth around the Thrusting Channel.

The circulation of Qi begins in the lower dan tien. The Sea of Qi is a storage container or cauldron of Qi energy. Sifu called it our Qi bank account. By breathing into the lower dan tien in this practice we accumulate Qi energy. This Field of Elixir is the source of meridian Qi, created by the energy we receive from earth, heaven, and our breath.

As my Sifu explained it, Circulation of Light practice begins with a few breaths, filling the Sea of Qi as if it were a big cauldron or chalice. The lower dan tien fills up with Qi and spills over into the perineum (Yin Confluence) and then flows down into the tailbone area which is the beginning of the Governing Channel. With the inhale, the ball of light moves up your back strengthening your spine. It moves through the Ming Men and into the upper dan tien where it is refined and transformed into spiritual vitality. The energy moves up over the crown of your head (Hundred Confluence) and down through your forehead and the Third Eye.

Then the Qi flows through the tongue which connects the yang Governing Channel with the yin Conceptual Channel. The Qi is guided down the front of the body, with the exhale. It moves through the middle dan tien and your heart and then returns to the lower dan tien. As the Qi descends, it nourishes all the organs.

Qi always works with prevailing energy conditions, to balance and restore equilibrium. If we are tired it perks us up. If we are anxious, it calms us down. This powerful practice strengthens and relaxes our body bringing harmony to the entire system. It is one of the oldest practices known, possibly five thousand years old.

This is a powerful practice. Toxins and debris in the body can be released causing reactions of dizziness, headaches, uncomfortable emotional states, and other symptoms. If you experience these reactions, stop, rest, hydrate and consult an experienced teacher.

Practice Form Seventeen: Circulation of Light

In the stance of Wuji, after connecting to heaven, earth, and your breath, you can begin the Circulation of Light.

To begin, place your tongue at the roof of your mouth. Visualize your breath energy as a ball of radiant light filling the lower dan tien, the Sea of Qi. When you feel there is enough energy, let the energy ball, spill over and sink down to your perineum. Feel the ball of light move to the bottom of your spine, the coccyx. Then with an inhale, let the Qi rise up your back. With a long inhale, allow your mind's attention to follow the surge of energy as it moves up your spine. The energy moves up over the crown of your head, and down through your forehead to the tongue. With the exhale, the Qi softly flows down through the Conceptual Channel. It brings nourishing Qi to the front of the body and all your organs. The ball of light again fills the lower Field of Elixir with Qi.

In many Qigong exercises, in stillness practices or where the movements and steps are repetitious, you can use the micro-cosmic breath. You can follow your breath, paced at the rate of your natural comfort.

Walking Meditation with Prayer Beads

Sifu taught us many meditation forms. One evening, in the upper room at the Sonoma school, he had us practice centering our mind on one object. We would sit in a circle with a candle in the center and focus our mind and breath on the candle. We would also do chanting. Sometimes, we walked in procession around the room close to the walls, making a big square with special footwork on the corners to make the flow seamless and graceful. We would usually go in a clockwise direction, so the last step on one wall would be with the left foot, allowing the right foot to easily swing around to start the 90-degree angle setting the new direction.

Sometimes Sifu would lead us in chanting the mantra to Kuan Yin in Chinese. He expected us to follow the chant with him 108 times. "Namo, Tai Chi, Tai Pi. Kuan Shih Yin, Pusa!" He would lead us in a slow walk around the room and we would follow repeating the strange sounds to the best of our ability. His dark shiny prayer beads moved through his graceful fingers one at a time for each time we said the chant. There was a big bead at the end of the strand with a tassel to mark the 108th bead. As I invited the Goddess within myself to listen and hear my own heart, I experienced a peaceful feeling.

It's difficult for me to find the time for a regular meditation practice. When I wake up in the morning, I find myself ruminating and obsessing. I realized if I took time right then and meditated right there in bed for a few minutes, then everything would straighten itself out.

I loved Tai Chi the first time I saw it, and yet it has been difficult for me to find the time and the will to practice.

When I was a student, I often met with my classmates and that inspired me to keep practicing. The group energy held and carried me. I needed other people to do the form with, so I began teaching. I teach Qigong and Tai Chi several times a week.

It is often easier to practice with a group. Buddhists speak of "spiritual friendship" and having a community or sangha where people can meditate together. When I moved from the farm, I found a sangha in Cloverdale that meets weekly.

Maturity

After the Farm

I left the Mendocino farm, after twenty years, because of irreconcilable differences with my partner Sue. This also meant we had to dissolve our ceramic business. I tried for years to make our relationship work. I realized it had reached its natural end. I learned being in harmony may mean withdrawing and reconnecting somewhere else.

My daughter moved two hundred miles to the north to live with her father and go to college. I started taking care of a hundred-year-old woman who had suffered a stroke and was in a wheelchair. I stayed with her four nights and three days a week. I continued my farm duties and hired a milkmaid who also fed the chickens, rabbits, and my cat on the days I was away doing homecare. On my days on the farm, I made cheese for sale and tended a small garden.

I was teaching two Qigong and Tai Chi classes a week and I practiced on my own and did daily chanting to help with my stress.

Life and PYNK in Cloverdale

One rainy winter I realized I was exhausted by traveling back and forth to work and trying to live in two places. The demands of taking care of the farm got to be too much. I just couldn't bring myself to slaughter one more rabbit. I finally made the decision to let go of the farm after losing my favorite goat to illness. I sold or gave away the rest of the animals.

In 1997 I bought a ranch style two-bedroom home on a half-acre in Cloverdale. The property used to be a small parcel out of town, but as the town grew it was now a larger parcel within the city limits. It had a nice orchard. I could pick fruit just about any day of the year from the first fruits of the loquats in May, to winter Navel Oranges edible from January to May. The persimmons could last into November. I canned peaches, apricots, and applesauce.

I made a Tai Chi circle on the SW corner in the back yard, planting black bamboo to the north. My new land partner built me a Kuan, a tea house temple to the east of the Tai Chi circle. I call it my Qigong hospital. It's a platform with six poles holding up a coarsely shingled cedar roof. It has a comfortable cot and a cushioned chair. A cupboarded altar holds a bell and an incense pot. When it rains, I can do Qigong under the cover of the roof.

I continued my home care work with several agencies and IHSS, a state sponsored program for low-income people. I designed an organization in 2011 for independent home care workers. This allows us to have a community of support and we are able to network and make teams to give consistent, quality care to our local seniors. We call our program Local Care for Local Elders and have about twenty-five members who meet monthly at the Senior Center to improve our skills, share our concerns, and help support each other in our work. We've helped over a hundred people in our community to be able to live and die in their own homes.

When I moved to Cloverdale, I kept my school's name, Po Yun Nei Kuan, White Cloud Women's Temple School. I teach Qigong and Tai Chi classes in my back yard, at the local Parkpoint health club, the Senior Center, and at the lodge in the new Del Webb senior housing that was built next door in the old Moulton Vineyard.

Return to the Uncarved Block

I am grateful to be here, and I still get anxious and depressed. It seems to be my nature, but mostly I am content when I return to my center. Following the advice of the old master Lao Tzu, I return to the state of the uncarved block, a place of nothingness, of Wuji. This is where creative possibilities arise for me.

I feel blessed that I can make a living with the work I love. I call my professions, of teaching Chinese internal martial arts and creating ceramics, my Double Happiness. Double Happiness is a popular character in Chinese calligraphy, usually a wish for the newly married. This is the blessing I receive from my work teaching Tai Chi and creating with clay.

Both arts require a return to stillness, to the empty space of Wuji. In the practice of Wuji meditation, as I focus on my present breath, I accept the plainness of my being, just as I am, knots and all. I wait. I watch the energies and thoughts come and go, the worries, the angers. I notice and listen to the concerns, but I don't react. I wait in stillness, re-centering into the fullness of my being like a pot centered on a potter's wheel, spinning in balance. The stability at my center enables the creative edge to be raised up with the even upward pressure, an invisible force of condensing and centering. Focusing on my breath, balancing around my center, finding the movement in the stillness and the stillness in the movement, are necessary qualities for both Tai Chi and throwing clay pots on a wheel.

Artists allow the creative process to flow through their being and be expressed. They become a conduit for creative energy, using their invisible desires and evolving consciousness for creative action. They return to what the

Taoists call the Uncarved Block: fresh, uncut, but full of creative potential.

"Do nothing, and nothing is undone," is a theme of the Tao Te Ching which promotes Wu Wei or non-action. It states, "The Way never acts, yet nothing is left undone."

The nameless uncarved block
Is but freedom from desire,
And if I cease to desire and remain still,
The empire will be at peace of its own accord.

Chapter 37 Tao te Ching

When we return to the state of nothingness, empty, listening to our breath, we return to the "uncarved block." We are open and fresh, ready to receive the Qi.

In the emptiness of returning, we find our intimate connection to everything around us. We feel the loving light in our heart, and the nurturing power of nature. In stillness our consciousness can encompass an awareness of a larger picture and the harmony of cause and effect. As we take our place in the oneness of our humanity, we know the peace of understanding. Not doing, just being, we allow the Qi to unfold naturally as we follow our breath.

Above, Below, Within

A calling in three parts

All Hail to Thee, All That is Above

Left arm raised to touch the sky
We call to all that soar and fly
Great winged ones – cranes, owl and dove
Dance among the clouds above
With drifting puff of changing shapes
We gaze, reflect, and scry our fates

The sky, the star, the moon and sun
transmit that we are All and None.
A part of the multi-verse we are,
Water, air, earth and fiery star
Through our breath, earth's atmosphere,
We plunge on down through shadowed fear.

We call you now in this time of peril.

All Hail to Thee, All That is Below

Right arm reaching to touch the earth
This is the hallowed place of birth
The topmost level, fairy-blessed
We journey inward, earth compressed,
The weight of gravity, strata of rock
Water flows through channeled loch

Sacred doors open to the fire within
Our bodies, crucibles, filled to the brim,

Swimming through dirt, we feel ourselves rise
Knowing for earth there's no compromise
Roots drinking water, feeding off dirt
We enter our garden, our will to assert

We call you now in this time of peril

All Hail to Thee, All That is Within

Both arms gather the All That Is
Hands crossed upon the heart that gives
Informing self of the work at hand
Intention and magick gives grace to the land
The body is upright, the center, the tree
The pillar that stands, it's you and it's me.

Up from our roots, through our center, to sky
Connecting what is from below to on high
Our body, a temple, a column of prayer
Offers our magic into the air
Words travel forth on the air that we breathe
The flame that makes change is what we believe.
Love flows through our hearts, a tear-sweetened stream
Axis Mundi, envisioned, we realize the dream.

We call you now in this time of peril,
And in this moment of grace.

Poem by, Marylyn Motherbear Scott

THE END

THE PYNK QIGONG FORM

Development of PYNK Qigong

The development of PYNK Qigong came from the fundamental principles that I learned over thirty years of training and teaching. The PYNK Qigong Form is considered a medical qigong form, concentrating on health not martial arts. The form massages every joint and organ of the body. It increases range of motion, balance and flexibility. It also incorporates the stimulation of specific acupuncture points to heal and harmonize the whole body. It is a daily practice for good health and can be a warm up for Tai Chi. The form is done from a standing position which helps bone density strength, although many movements can be adapted to a sitting position.

The name PYNK came from the name of my school Po Yun Nei Kuan which means White Cloud Women's Temple School which I established in the hills and clouds of Mendocino County in 1980. It was the northern reflection of Lung Lu Shan Tzu The Dragon Tiger Mountain Temple School of my Sifu's, which was in the county to the south,

269

as it is in China. I wanted to honor the root of my beloved practice from China and my fascination and identification with clouds. Clouds float through heaven and give us nourishing rain for life, as qigong gives nourishment to our body, which is the temple of our mind and spirit.

PYNK Qigong is not meant for women only. The benefits of health can be enjoyed by all people. I gladly and eagerly share this gift of health, and deeper relationship to self and all life.

The form begins with Wuji meditation to connect the practitioner with the Three Powers of earth, sky and human energy. This Wuji or Simple Standing posture aligns the body into softness so qi energy flows freely because the body is relaxed and in balance. The form continues with massaging the body with ROM (Range of Motion) circles and movements that loosen tight areas. It includes stimulating acupuncture points which increase qi flow to harmonize and heal organs and systems. PYNK Qigong is internal work based on bringing the mind's loving attention into the body.

Qigong movements help cleanse the body of toxins. Motion helps the heart push the blood to reach every cell delivering the oxygen and nutrients the body needs. It helps cleanse the blood by massaging and supporting the function of the kidneys, the liver, and the lungs. Movement helps lymph to flow boosting the immune system. The treatment involves moving every joint and organ of the body. It massages and relaxes the muscles relieving tension and pain. The gentle movements and relaxation techniques of qigong improve and harmonize organ and gland function.

PYNK Qigong is a treatment that you give yourself for health and relaxation in about twenty to forty minutes. If the practitioner is ill, weak, or has an injury, the form can be modified and adapted. Start with less movement and increase the number of repetitions of specific exercises to get stronger as your comfort level allows. You can start with a few rotations of the joints and increase the ROM as your joints get stronger and more flexible. Spend more time on the stillness practices teaching your body to relax and heal.

Stillness practice is often the most difficult for people. "Not doing" is counter intuitive in our western culture. We value being busy. Standing in meditation challenges us both physically and psychologically. We notice issues like chronic pain. Maybe an old rage we thought was gone shows up in angry thoughts or deep sadness. Fears, old injuries, boredom and anxiety can all come to our attention when we stand in stillness. Through the power of staying still we allow the breath and relaxation techniques to melt and release the painful tight places whether the pain is physical, emotional or mental. When we soften and maintain curiosity, we can explore and heal our discomfort through the loving attention of our mind and the ability of the breath to restore balance and harmony.

Qigong and Tai Chi require full participation by the practitioner. It is not a passive treatment. It is not something someone else does for you. The patient is also the healer. It takes work and active attention to cultivate the channels of qi to open and flow. The relaxation we achieve in qigong is not limp but active alignment of the body. The whole person is engaged.

The word "gong" in qigong means work accomplished or skill that requires time and effort. The gong is accumulated through daily discipline not sporadic practice. Daily practice, even for short periods of time, creates the powerful reservoir of qi through the accumulation of gong. Qigong supports your body and clears your mind, so you have the ability to do what you want. The unnecessary is discarded and true value is retained.

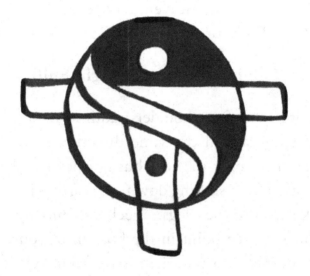

The logo for PYNK Qigong represents
the Tai Chi Symbol
And the manifestation of our human form
Dancing the Tai Chi with Choice
Image by Janet Seaforth

PYNK Qigong Practice

Simu Janet Seaforth, Po Yun Nei Kuan

Wuji: Not Doing, State of Emptiness,
Standing meditation
Alignment with Three Powers,
Earth, Heaven, Humanity
Whole Body Breathing, Yin/Yang awareness,

Solid and Empty Weight Shift

Begin with your feet shoulder width apart and parallel, toes point forward in the same direction as your knees. Bend the knees over the toes but not beyond them. Feel the relaxation from sinking down into earth with the knees bent, like having "sea legs." Feel the Bubbling Spring, the Kidney Source point in the bottom of your feet as it connects deeply into the earth like a root. Appreciate all the earth gives, our food, our water, the air we breathe and beauty of nature. Feel the energy of the earth which is gravity. Gravity gives us the balance point. Gravity is the root of balance. "When the body is in perfect balance there is no strain on any part of it." Find this root, align your body with it and relax.

Feel your hips resting on your two strong soft legs. Feel the "basket of bones," your pelvic girdle that holds up the trunk of your body so your body and all its organs and parts can relax into alignment with your centerline. The shoulders are relaxing over the hips. The head lightly lifts up as the back of the neck lengthens upward. Feel as if you are being pulled up to heaven by a silver thread, dangling, like a plum-bob into the centerline of gravity. The centerline from heaven connects to the earth root of balance at the lower dan tien just below the navel.

"Feet stand on earth, head touches heaven." Now open the crown of your head and feel the big blue sky and beyond to all the stars and planets in our cosmos. Feel the radiant cosmic energy of the universe, the creative source that made all there is from the Big Bang billions of years ago. From nothing came something and the universe has been expanding ever since forming all that is seen and unseen. Feel the Power of Heaven. The universe is in us from the elements that are in our body created by stars in the furnace of their explosions. "The universe is in us, and we are in the universe." Feel the oneness of creation. Feel the electromagnetic energy that surrounds your body, a Torus Field of energy. Feel the Wei Chi, the protective energy that surrounds the body and is strengthened with awareness practice.

Bring your mind's attention to your breath, placing your hands on the lower dan tien, right hand first, left hand covering the right. Feel into the Third Power, the power of Humanity. Stand in Simple Standing posture, aligned, in a state of Wuji, Not Doing. Notice as you bring your attention to your breath you relax more deeply. Feel your whole-body breathing, as you inhale the belly expands slightly, as you exhale the belly contracts slightly. Breathe into any tight or painful places. Allow the breath to reharmonize the body with peaceful energy. Feel the movement in stillness. When you are ready, shift the weight of the body to the right foot. The knee is bent, ninety percent of the weight is on the right foot, the body is still in alignment. The shoulders are relaxing over the hips. The head is still lightly lifting up. Weight bearing increases bone density. After a few minutes shift your weight to the left leg for the same amount of time.

Begin moving meditation, shift the weight to your centerline with the inhale and to the solid foot or weight bearing foot with the exhale. Coordinate your breath with your movements, always inhaling to center and exhaling to the solid foot. Continue moving from side to side slowly and evenly without stopping. Feel the stillness in the movement. After a few repetitions, bring the body back to center and take a few breathes.

The Bow

Bring the feet together, hands drop down to the sides. We Say "Kuan Li," which means "merciful behavior." We are merciful to ourselves, to others and to nature itself. Bring the hands up at the sides, gathering qi from earth and sky and make a fist with the right hand and with the left hand cover the fist. This is a hand mudra called "Chain Link of Grace." Let the mudra float down the body like a pearl dropped into oil through all three dan tiens to the base. The hands naturally turn over with the backs of the hands on the bottom. Bow from the hips bringing the hands up to the upper dan tien with the arms extended. Extend your covered fist three times to acknowledge mind, body and spirit, and the others if you are in a group. When we practice alone, we usually face north to pay respect to the Great Unknown, to remind ourselves we always face the unknown.

If you are practicing with a group, it is good to work in a circle. Everyone is facing each other to acknowledge everyone's qi. Connecting your qi with everyone else's, creates a qi field. Bowing in and acknowledging each person's energy strengthens the healing potential through the qi field created by unified intention. In qigong we bring the mind's loving attention into the service of the body for health and happiness.

Massaging Circles and Stretches

After Wuji and our salutation we begin the basic qigong practice keeping our feet together, hands on our knees, for **knee circles** which gives our knees Range of Motion (ROM). Feel the movements in our knees, ankles, feet and the nice massage we give the bottoms of our feet. Continue in a gentle even flow.

After several repetitions before we reverse direction, we straighten the knees, make the back flat and **dangle**. Release the hips, drop the hands towards or on the ground and exhale to relax. Shake and wiggle a little to release tension. The weight of the upper body helps stretch muscles in the back of the legs by passive traction. The weight of the heavy head helps release neck tension through passive traction and more blood goes to the brain strengthening capillaries. Being upside down is good for the body. It is like a yoga head stand with less effort.

Come back to center and bring the hands back to rest on the knees reversing the knee circles. Make sure you do an equal number on each side. Pay attention to what is moving and what is still and relaxed. The elbows and shoulders remain relaxed, the Ming Men is open. Then straighten the knees, keep the back flat and release the hips one more time dropping the hands towards the ground with the exhale and a big sigh of release. Blow some air out of your mouth. As muscles relax you will often be able to have more flexibility and your hands can reach the ground.

While you are still dangling **stretch** to the left side opening the right waist and closing the left waist, keeping the hips forward. Feel the stretch and inhale back to center then stretch to the right side. This **opens and closes the waist** and moves the organs which helps keep them fresh by pushing out waste products and bringing in fresh blood. Come back to center take a breath exhaling stale energy into the ground through hands and feet. Unfurl your body coming up to centered standing, coming up one vertebra at a time.

Place feet shoulder width for **hip circles**, putting the hands on the hips, and move the hips around the axis in nice easy even hip circles. Feel the skeletal structure of the hips moving in ROM around the center line. Feel the hip joints and sacrum opening and closing increasing flexibility. Then bring the mind into the lower abdominal cavity and feel the massaging action supporting and cleansing the digestive, elimination, and reproductive systems as the movement pushes out stale energy and brings in fresh energy and blood. After massaging one way, reverse for a similar number of circles. Moving in circles is very relaxing and comforting to the body. It increases endorphin levels and supports the immune system.

Place your feet together for **waist circles**. Put your hands over the kidneys which are located about waist height at either side of the spine. Lift your upper abdominal cavity slightly to create more space. Massage upper abdominal organs through ROM circles. Feel into the liver and kidneys. As you move feel the closing and opening, the squeezing and releasing of the organs. This movement cleans them like a sponge, squeezing out the old energy and debris and bringing in fresh blood and qi. Pay attention to other organs of the upper abdominal area: the pancreas, spleen, stomach and upper intestines. Give appreciation and gratitude to all that your wonderful body does to keep you healthy and strong.

Swings Around the Axis

Place your feet shoulder width apart, lift the arms up at your sides at shoulder height led by the wrists. The wrists are held up the shoulders relax down. The posture is like a bird with its wings spread to dry. The waist turns. The lower dan tien located just below the navel is the source of the action. Movements in qigong and tai chi originate from this center of power. **Swing around the axis** of your body, look behind yourself at horizon level. The body follows the eyes and the arms swing out and fall against the hips. The feet stay grounded and the weight doesn't shift. Your whole body is engaged.

As soon as you feel your arms slapping against your hips turn your neck and look behind yourself to the other side. Swing back and forth loosely. Twist to the right and left. Fell the energy coming from the centerline and moving out to the hands. Move from the lower dan tien. The legs do the work. Keep your knees bent slightly as your body swings around your axis. This loosens the shoulder and twists the whole body as the spine gently turns. This is the first swing of three.

For the **second swing** bring one foot out in the direction of your eyes as you look behind. The arms swing in the same pattern as in the first swing. Additionally you lift and point your toe in the direction you are looking. The pivot is on the heels, the weight stays in center as you move around the axis like a child's top. This helps prevent falling as you train your feet to follow your eyes. Continue the swing side to side. Feel your body gently twisting from your feet to the top of your head. Feel the spiral energy coming up from the earth to the top of your head as you twist. Lead the movement from the lower dan tien, as if it was a search light looking right and left as you swing. This movement strengthens your ability to keep your balance while you are in motion. There's no muscle use in the arms. They are passive. Sifu Nam Singh says to pretend you have heavy bracelets on your wrists to help your arms swing out as you loosen your shoulders and elbows.

The **third swing** starts by coming back to center with your feet shoulder width apart. The feet move the same as the second swing, but the action of the arms creates a wringing action for the whole body. Bring your hands up to eye level or above your head with your palms facing each other. Whenever the palms face each other the Lao Gong points in the center of each palm can be energetically connected. This forms a Qi Ball. The Lao Gong points can be used for sending and receiving qi. Feel the energy between your palms as you cultivate the skill of sending and receiving qi.

Now throw the ball down in an arc as you turn, as you did in the second swing. Let the ball pop up over your head as look behind you. Throw the ball to arc down and pop up in front of the body and then to the other side in a continuous flow. Right toe out, turn right; right toe in come to center. Left toe out, turn left; left toe in come back to center. Swing back right, arms up right, throw the ball down and back up to center. Throw the ball down and swing back left, ball pops up over your head and as you throw it down again it swings back up to center. The weight of the wrists and arms powers the movement. There is little effort as you swing around your axis. Th action of moving the arms up and down is relaxed. This opens and loosens the shoulder joints. The swinging action pumps and cleanses the lymph glands in the arm pits and helps to prevent breast cancer. The arms maintain a strong-arm shape because you are holding on to the qi ball. This shape is good for blocking in the martial arts. You use the force of momentum with little muscle strength. The movement is finished as you come back to center with the qi ball at eye level or above your head.

Harmonize with Qi

With your arms held above your head open your palms to the sky. Receive the heavenly original qi (Yuan Qi) and loving light through the Lao Gong points. Turn palms to focus and project qi to the top of the head to open the Bai Hui point. The Bai Hui is the top of the Thrusting Channel. The Thrusting Channel is a central column of energy that goes all the way down to the perineum connecting all three dan tiens in the head, heart and belly. Feel Yuan Qi enter the body and fill this central channel.

Now feel your body surrounded by loving light. Feel this light filling your body's energy field. Sense the electromagnetic field of energy that surrounds you. You can also feel the Wei Qi, the protective invisible shield around your body. Imagine your body surrounded by light. Bring any color into your mind that feels healing and strengthening. This takes about three breaths, but you may keep this position as long as you want.

Slowly bring your palms down your body as you project the loving light of qi from the palms of your hands to harmonize every cell, tissue, and organ of your body. This is a qi treatment you give yourself. The loving light of qi, heals and integrates all parts of the body. Feel the loving light of qi all the way from the top of your head to your feet. Take a deep breath and soak it in.

You can say Haola! which means, "All is well!" The body wants to do the mind's bidding. Affirmations give the body a chance to move in the direction of wellness and healing.

More Massaging Circles

Now the shoulders are loose and relaxed and ready for **shoulder ROM**. Bring the shoulders forward and up with the inhale, and back and down with the exhale for shoulder circles back. After a few rotations, reverse to shoulder circles forward. Inhale as the shoulders come up and forward and exhale as they drop down and back. Feel the opening and closing of the clavicle in the front and the scapula in the back as you make the rotations. Bring the shoulders into harmony with each other, release shoulder tension. Feel the deep massage you are giving yourself. Notice the movement of the thoracic cavity, ribs, lungs, heart. Breathe deeply to exercise the lungs. To finish do one shoulder circle back to open the chest.

Connecting to the Three Treasures, Shen, Jing and Qi

Feel centered and relaxed as you give yourself a feather massage dragging your finger-tips across your chest to open the heart center, the middle dan tien. Now in a relaxed state put the tip of the middle finger which is at the end of the pericardium meridian, on the lower sternum, to connect to the **Shen energy that lives in your heart and mind.**

The shen is called the Immortal Spirit, the Deathless, the Knower, the Everlasting. **It is your evolving consciousness** that is uniquely you and yet connected with the universal consciousness and all of creation. Feel this energy like a wave in the ocean of qi, unique and yet connected. Feel into your breathing, re-membering the energy in the mind and heart which is beyond the body and the thinking mind. The shen energy can direct the mind. It is a guide to our utmost truth. It is your true self.

Stimulate the Points

Kidneys

Make an eagle's beak with the right hand bringing the fingers and thumb together. Use this to tap the upper sternum which **stimulates the thymus gland.** The thymus is located under the sternum and makes the **T-cells** that flow through the blood and take out pathogens, viruses and cancer cells from the entire body. Give you body permission to be disease free.

Use the tips of your fingers to rub little circles into the **Kidney-27** point, to harmonize the waters of the body, and our **Jing energy**. This point is **a toxic release point** in a little hollow located below the clavicle on either side of the sternum. Stimulation of this point harmonizes the waters of the body, cleansing out the toxins. Drink water after your session if you stimulate this point to help flush out toxins.

Lungs

Move your fingers to the outside of your clavicle and under it, by the shoulder. Rub up and down to stimulate the lung points 1 and 2. They are only about an inch apart. Rub with the thumb or index and middle fingers if that's easier. Breathe deeply to **stimulate and cleanse the lungs.** Know you are breathing with all the plants and animals on this planet, sharing oxygen and carbon dioxide. Our breath energy is interconnected with all life on this planet. This is the **Treasure of Qi, our Life Breath energy.**

Shamen Shake

Shake your body moving organically, in the moment, subconsciously. **Shake out tension**. Make sounds if you like releasing tensions, groan, sigh, shout. Stamp your feet if you feel like it. Then tighten up for a few moments and then relax.

Notice yin and yang energy

Relax your body into the **soft stillness** of aligned posture so the energy can flow freely. Then make fists with the arms extended horizontally in front of your body. **Extend and contract your fingers,** keeping your shoulders relaxed as you pump your hands. Feel the active or yang quality of your hands while keeping the yin, soft, relaxed quality of your body.

Rubs

Make fists and with the mouth of the fist, (index finger and thumb side) rub the **kidneys,** either side of the spine at waist level. Nourish and support your kidneys by massaging the **Ming Men.** Move up to your **adrenal glands** which sit on top of your kidneys. Exhale to release tension. Move the fists down the back into the lower back to **rub out any low back tension** with your knuckles. Finally rub the end of the tailbone with your fingertips to stimulate the spinal fluid to pump up the spinal cord and into your brain to lubricate and nourish your **central nervous system.**

Spiral to Heaven

Place your hands on your hips with your feet shoulder width apart and root down. From the tailbone lift up and lengthen the spine putting space between the vertebrae, stretching up as if the head were touching the sky. Relax your arms and hands at your sides. Then make little head circles loosening up the neck as you stretch the spine. This is a qigong movement called Spiraling to Heaven. After a few rotations reverse and circle the other way. Feel a spiral of energy connecting you to the cosmos.

Moving the Atlas and Axis Vertebrae

Come back to center with an erect body making sure your head and shoulders are aligned. Drop your ear to your left shoulder, exhale and relax. Inhale, rotate your neck and head a quarter turn to bring your chin to that shoulder. This moves the atlas and axis vertebrae at the top of the spine. Inhale as you return to center. Do the same thing on the other side. **Exhale ear to shoulder, inhale chin to shoulder**, exhale ear to shoulder, inhale up to center.

Stretch Neck and Circle Head

The feet are grounded, the knees are bent. From a centered position drop your chin to your chest and relax your jaw. Tilt the head back and bring your face up to face the sky.

Move your eyes in different directions; back and forth, up and down. Center your eyes and drop your chin to your chest. Consciously relax your shoulders, elbows, wrists and hands. Let any unwanted tension release through the bottoms of your feet into the earth with a big exhale. One more time bring the face to the sky and make circles with your eyes both ways in even circles for good eye health. Return to center and drop the chin to the chest and make large head rotations for ROM of your neck. As the head rolls around, lean back as the head goes back to protect your neck vertebrae. When you get your chin back to your chest reverse direction letting any tension drift away.

Feel the Qi

Come back to center, rotate your wrists to open with the palms forward. Arms slightly outstretched. Feel the qi flowing through your body. Your whole body is alert but relaxed. Feel the inner smile deep inside. Feel the natural state of contentment. Breathe a few breathes in enjoyment.

Articulate the fingers into fists

Bring your fists in front of your shoulders, elbows in to open the scapula in the back, turn your wrists so your fists face out. Articulate your fingers, one finger at a time. Opening and closing the fists. Begin with the little fingers out, then the ring finger, the middle finger, the index finger, and thumb until your hands are open. Then starting with the little fingers closing in, followed with the ring finger, middle finger, index finger and thumb until you have made fists again. Opening and closing the fists in repetition to loosen the hands and keep then fingers supple. The Chinese say, "The hinges on a gate that is used often do not rust."

Celestial Drumming

Celestial Drumming is a qigong form to stimulate deep into the body's endocrine system. The endocrine system is made of glands which secrete hormones the body needs. Secretions from the pancreas balance blood-sugar levels. The thyroid gland controls metabolism and our growth and development. The adrenal glands give us our fight or flight hormones and balances fluid levels. The **endocrine system** is the body's own natural pharmacy giving the body what it needs to be in homeostasis and harmony.

Place the heel of your palm over your ears to block out outside sounds. Flick your middle finger off your index finger at the back of your head. You will hear a clicking sound, a "drumming" into your head. With your intention send the qi energy to the center of the brain to the pituitary gland, which is the master gland for the endocrine system. Imagine your entire endocrine system being harmonized with qi. Concentrate on your own pharmacy deep inside your body. Allow your body to refresh itself. Haola! After about thirty-two clicks, pop the hands off the ears and feel the harmony.

Balance Work

Crane Flies: Feet are shoulder width apart, your arms at your sides. Inhale and bring the left foot into cat stance. Your weight stabilizes on your right foot as your wrists rise to shoulder level. The elbows are relaxing down with the wrists up and hands relaxed, like the wings of a bird. Exhale and float your hands down in front of your body. Inhale lifting your hands up to the sides as before. Simultaneously bring your left knee up. Your left foot is at the level of your right knee. Crane Stands on One Leg. Exhale while your hands and foot float down to beginning position. Inhale rise your arms up over your head until the back of your hands touch. Your knee again rises up to about waist level, Crane Spreads Wings. Exhale as you lower the arms and reach out with your left foot to the original shoulder width. Touch down with your toe follow with the heel, sink down and move your weight to your left foot. With the inhale bring the right toe into a cat stance as you lift your wrists again to shoulder height. Repeat the three movements on each side until you feel a continuous flow like a great crane flying. Finally come back to center, inhale as you bring your hands to your lower dan tien right hand first, left hand cover. Breathe a few breathes and harmonize with qi.

Closing

Bow out to close the Qi Field in gratitude. Say Kuan Li, (Merciful Behavior) to yourself, to others in the circle. And thank all teachers that have given us these healing forms through many centuries.

Finally cross your hands over your heart with a commitment to give yourself some Qi Love every day.

GLOSSARY

Acupuncturists Traditional Chinese Medicine practitioners who work with specific Qi points where the Qi is close to the surface of the skin. These points are found along the meridians of the body. The acupuncturist places needles at specific points to help Qi flow and harmonize the body and its organs.

Animal Frolics are Qigong exercises attributed to the famous acupuncturist and surgeon Hua Tua, who lived about 2000 years ago in the Han Dynasty. He designed exercises to mimic the movements and strengths of five animals, tiger, bear, deer, monkey and crane. These coincide with the five vital organs of the body, lung, kidney, liver, heart, and spleen. The practices stimulate the specific organ's meridians.

Ba Gua or Eight Directions is not simply points on a compass, but a philosophy of how creation unfolds. The development of the Ba Gua created a number system that could describe the qualities of Heaven, Earth, and Humanity. The ancient Chinese believed that Creation starts with the Great Tao which is undifferentiated and unknowable. Differentiation started with the Tai Chi. What is one becomes two, the opposing forces of yin and yang. From these forces the rest of creation is formed through the Eight Directions, as distribution of yin yang energy forms all the various possibilities. Through the Ba Gua, the story of creation and culture came alive.

Baihui Acupuncture point on the top of the head meaning "hundred meeting." It opens to the Cosmos.

Big Bang beginning of creation of our universe about 13.7 billion years ago. Out of nothing came something. The elements that are in our body were made in the stars of heaven. The universe is literally in us, as we are in the universe. A state of grace is developed when we can maintain our ability to stay in the presence of this awareness.

Bodhidharma or Daruma was a Buddhist monk from India who came to the palace of Emperor Wu and assisted him with the translations of the Buddhist Sanskrit. Bodhidharma told Emperor Wu that he gained no merit in granting the Shaolin temple. He advocated that it was only by his own internal process of mind that he would reach Nirvana, not by good deeds. Bodhidharma left the palace and made his way to the Young Forest Shaolin Temple monastery.

Bodhisattva is one who refuses, or delays, going to heaven until all suffering on earth has ended. Kuan yin is known as a bodhisattva.

Circulation of Light see Micro-Cosmic orbit.

Chain Link of Grace. The mudra Chain link of Grace is made up of the Boxer and the Scholar, with a right hand fist and a cover of the fist with our left hand.

Chang San Feng The founder of Tai Chi Chuan He was a Taoist monk, scholar, and warrior in the time of the Mongol invasion of China in the thirteenth century, born on the revered mountain Wudang at the end of the Sung Dynasty in April of 1247.

Chen Man Ching a Grand Master of Tai Chi Chuan. His name is sometimes spelled Jan Man Ching. Grand Master of Tai Chi Chuan.

Chuan means fist. It is known as the fist of self-containment, it signifies refusing to be a victim and taking responsibility for our life.

Confucius also known as Kong Qiu or K'ung Fu-tzu, 551–479 BC. He is a revered teacher and philosopher emphasizing proper behavior and ritual, which is reflected in the family patterns of the Eight Directions, of the Ba Gua.

Dan tian, are three areas in the body of powerful energy fields, called the fields of elixir. Lower dan tien is called the Sea of Qi, just below the navel. Middle dan tien is at the heart. Upper dan tien is in the head. The lower dan tien is called the Qi bank account. Daily practice keeps Qi in the Sea of Qi reservoir to be used when you need it.

Eagles Beak or Mantis Hand gathers up energy with the fingers together pointing down to the earth and the wrist bends up towards heaven. The high bend of the wrist is seen as a weapon like a fist or an elbow. It is also used as a hook to trap, block and parry an opponent.

Feng Shui means "wind-water." Feng-Shui is used to keep evil spirits away and increase good Qi. It uses what is called the Magic Square, based on the Later Heaven Model of the Ba Gua to illustrate this movement. Feng Shui works to balance energy to achieve greater productivity, happiness, and health in structures as homes, offices, grave sites, and gardens.

Five Elements see Wu Xing

Five Essential Qualities are slowness, evenness, calmness, clarity, and balance. They are the qualities exemplified in the practice of Tai Chi.

Fuxi is credited with inventing the Ba Gua from the images on a tortoise's back. He lived in Henan province about 4,000 years ago and proclaimed himself as the first monarch. His Kingdom extending to the east coast in the first dynasty called the Xia (Hsia).

Hsing-i or Xing Yi Quan means Form-Intention Fist or Shape-Will Fist. It refers to the ability of the mind to create an idea and project it into the body. It is considered the most yang of the internal arts.

Hui Tuo, was a great physician credited with creating several forms of Qigong that are well documented from about 2000 years ago, including the classic Animal Frolics and the Ba Duan Jing or Eight Brocades.

Huiyin acupuncture point called Yin Convergence. It is located at the perineum the bottom of the Thrusting Channel.

Hun or soul according to TCM is the part of our consciousness that contains our desires, plans, dreams, and imagination. At night it gives us our dreams as the blood collects and is filtered by the liver when we are sleeping. The hun is thought to reside in the liver. In the day, our hun or soul looks out through our eyes. The eyes are the window to the soul. Taoists paid close attention to their dreams to increase their understanding of the messages from heaven. Our hun and our shen are both parts of our consciousness.

I Ching or Yi Jing is a book of philosophy of how yin and yang play out their infinite combinations. It is based on the Eight Direction arranged in basic trigrams which combine to form the 64 hexagrams which represent the archetypal situations in human life. The I Ching, or Book of Changes, developed over millennia. From its beginning the I Ching has been used as an oracle. People still consult the I Ching to divine their fate and seek knowledge for the best action.

Jade Emperor is the God of Heaven, or Mr. Heaven, known as Yu Huang or Yu Di. He named the animals in the twelve-year cycle of Chinese New Year.

Jing is one of the Three Treasures. It is the consolidation of Qi into solid form. It is a yin energy associated with water. According to Traditional Chinese Medicine we inherit Jing from our ancestors. It is associated with our DNA or inherited Qi. In Chinese Traditional Medicine the Jing is stored in the Ming Men, the Gate of Life which is associated with the kidneys. Through Qigong practice we protect, conserve, and enhance our Jing energy.

Kuan Li is a salute that means, "merciful behavior." It is used when we bow, to pay respect and honor to who we truly are, to respect others in the group and their uniqueness and finally we pay respect to nature itself and seek through understanding to be in harmony with Her.

Kuan Yin is commonly known as the Goddess of Fearless Compassion or the Goddess of Mercy and "She who hears the cries of the world." She is the most beloved Goddess of the Chinese.

Li is behavior, or patterns of behavior. It is understood as the natural growth patterns of creation, from the grains and knots in wood and jade, to the evolutionary patterns found in DNA. Each living organism is unique and has its own natural unfolding. Li is the structure through which energy moves. It is the pattern energy uses to create form. Li is the "implicate order" we observe in the manifestations of Qi.

Lo Pan, or Luo Pan is an elaborate and mysterious instrument using the compass of the Ba Gua. It is primarily used in the practice of Feng Shui. It was designed about two thousand years ago. Lo means a net that encompasses everything, pan means utensil or plate. It symbolizes the union of Heaven and Earth and the electromagnetic field that holds all matter together. A real compass with a magnetized needle in the center pointed south, the direction of Heaven. The Lo Pan is a complex system with concentric circles of information. The yin/yang symbol is in the center as energy moves out it includes the Five Elements, the Eight Directions, and twelve animal signs of the Chinese zodiac.

Lunar New Year. Following the cycles of the moon, the Chinese created their calendar. The moon, according to the Chinese, belongs to the Earth. The lunar calendar has Ten Heavenly Stems which correlate to the Five Elements and Twelve Earthly Branches, which are associated with the twelve animals of the Chinese zodiac.

Magic Square is a system which divides a square into nine parts of three by three. The order has a specific arrangement where the numbers of any line of three add up to fifteen. The numbering system creates a path of Qi which is powerful and considered magical.

Mandate of Heaven meant an emperor was sufficiently virtuous to rule. If he didn't fulfill his obligations, then he lost the Mandate and the right to be emperor.

Meditation is a practice of sitting standing or laying in stillness as we let our thoughts float through without attachment or aversion, being open to the eternal present.

Meridian Qi runs through our bodies along invisible pathways called channels or meridians. The meridians pass through numerous acupuncture points. Opening the flow of Qi through the meridians is a primary practice in Qigong.

Micro-Cosmic orbit is a breathing exercise, where the Qi up your back through the Governing Channel, the major yang meridian, and down the front of your body, the Conceptual Channel, the major yin meridian. It is also called Circulation of Light.

Ming Men is an acupressure point called the Gate of Life where we enter the earth plane.

Nei Jing, The Inner Canon is the oldest book of Traditional Chinese Medicine. It was written over 2000 years ago. It says: "The Meridians move Qi and Blood, regulate Yin and Yang, moisten the tendons and bones, and benefit the joints."

Mudra is a specific hand position for energy cultivation.

New year's almanac The Chinese almanac was carried to their destinations throughout the country on sedan chairs, placed on pedestals, and greeted with prostrations and a salute of guns on New Year's Day. The Book of Records contains notices given by the Perfect Emperor Yao in 2254 BCE to his astronomers commanding them to ascertain the solstices and equinoxes so the farmer might know when to plant.

Nu Wa is the creation Goddess. She is depicted in paintings and sculptures from the great art of the Tang Dynasty with her consort the first king of the Chinese people, **Fuxi.** This may signify the time when the institution of marriage was created. The two are depicted with their lower bodies as two snakes intertwined like a caduceus. In their hands they hold a compass and a carpenter's square. They are considered the architects of the Chinese people, their culture, and the ancestors of humankind.

PAWMA Pacific Association of Women in the Martial Arts a training association for women with annual camps from Seattle to Los Angeles.

Peng energy is a yang energy. Peng energy fills the area around the body and arms like filling up a big balloon. In I Chuan standing method the arms are extended, forming a circle to increase expansive, internal force or peng energy.

Po Yun Nei Kuan, PYNK, White Cloud Women's Temple School is the name of my Qigong Tai Chi Chuan school.

Postnatal Qi is the Qi we receive after birth. We can destroy or protect it, depending on our lifestyle and environment. Qigong helps cultivate our Postnatal Qi.

Primal Qi is the stuff like quanta that makes up everything. It is a balance of yin and yang in constant exchange. When the Qi condenses it makes form, when it disperses it returns to energy. It is like the interchange of matter and energy in the study of physics.

Primordial spirit or Yuan Qi. It is the guiding light that governs the powers of creation, the master architect of every atom and molecule, star, and planet in the ever-expanding temple of the manifest universe. It is the infinite ocean of consciousness from which the eternal spirit of each individual springs. As the transcendent mind of the universe, primordial spirit is the source of wisdom, compassion, and all spiritual virtue.

Push Hands is partner work in Tai Chi Chuan and Chinese martial arts.

Qi is the energy that makes up everything in our universe. It is like the quanta in physics and chemistry. The quanta is the minimum value of a physical property involved in an interaction. Qi is the vibrating energy like electricity that has an on and off quality, or yin/yang aspect. Qi is life force or vital energy in everybody and thing.

Qi is breath, or life breath energy. Qi is made of yin and yang. Our inhale breath is yin, and the outgoing breath or exhale is yang.

Qi Ball The palms often connect energetically through the Lao Gong points. This forms a Qi ball of energy.

Reiki is a popular Japanese healing system. Reiki is made up of two words. Rei is defined as: universal life energy, spiritual consciousness and all knowing. Rei is like the Chinese Yuan Qi or primal Qi energy. Ki in Japanese is like Qi in Chinese. It is breath, life force and vital radiant energy. The Japanese characters differ from the Chinese as the symbol is rain instead of steam. The Reiki practitioner or master is a conduit for healing Ki or Qi.

Sangha is a community of people that come together to meditate, usually Buddhist practitioners. We take "refuge" in the sangha to be free of danger, pursuit, or trouble.

Shaolin means Monastery in the forest or woods. The Shaolin Temple is renowned as the birthplace of the Chinese martial arts. It's founder, Batuo, means "man with consciousness."

Shen is one of the Three Treasures. It is associated with fire. It lives in our heart and mind and is referred to as the Immortal Spirit sometimes called the Eternal or the Deathless. It is our own individual evolving consciousness, which is unique and yet part of the Universal Consciousness. The Shen is the Knower, our true self. It is an energy which is beyond the body yet within the body. Shen is beyond the thinking mind and our emotions. It is an energy linked to eternity and universal consciousness.

Sifu a title for a male or female teacher of Qigong, Tai Chi Chuan and Chinese martial arts.

Simu a title which means "teacher mother" used for a female teacher of Chinese martial arts. It is often the title of the wife of a Sifu.

Snake and the Crane is a symbol, an icon in martial arts. Attributed to Chang San Feng who prayed and meditated and happened to see a fight between a snake and a crane. The snake is yin Earth. It lies close to the ground. It is a symbol of healing and herbal medicine. The crane is yang Heaven. It is seen as symbolizing longevity, immortality, happiness, and good fortune. It is the messenger of the Gods and intermediary between Heaven and Earth. It represents higher states of consciousness and the ability to travel to other worlds.

Sweet Dew or Heavenly Dew is a healing potion. The hours from 3:00 Am to 5:00 AM is known as the time of the "Sweet Dew". This is the best time for meditation. It is said that the dew has the potent power to heal. It also refers to the saliva that collects in the mouth during meditation.

Tai Chi means Supreme Ultimate. It is the name of the symbol of two fish swimming which represent yin yang in constant change.

Tai Chi Chuan is from the Wade-Giles translation, meaning Supreme Ultimate Fist. In modern pinyin translation it is written taijiquan. Tai translates as great. The ji is translated as pole or extreme, so taiji represents perfect balance and harmony with duality, but the word or character for Chi or Qi is absent. Forty years ago, Qigong was spelled Chi Kung or Chi Gung.

Tao is translated as The Way. Tao produced the natural order, which gives rise to the constant changes made by the play of yin and yang. The symbol for yin-yang is called the Tai Chi. It depicts two fish swimming within a circle of unity.

Taoism or Daoism It is an ancient study of being in harmony with nature. The Taoists describe the universe coming into being from nothing. Out of Wuji comes Tai Chi, "out of nothing came something,". The great void of Wuji created Tao which created Tai Chi. The great Tao is called The Way. The Way is the order of the universe and its creation. It's how things work.

Tao Te Ching, the oldest book of Taoism. It means The Way and its Power. Lao Tzu is the author. Lao Tzu mean "old man" and it could have been a compilation of many wise writers.

Te means virtue. It represents the inherent power of love and truth within us. Te is an inborn quality and the true original nature of humankind. The Chinese character for Te is a combination of the ideograms for a simplified foot combined with the modified characters for "true" and "heart." It is this true heart that upholds the Te.

Three Powers are called San Tsai. They are Heaven, Earth, and Humanity. They are fundamental to any Qigong practice.

Three Treasures or San Bao. They are three major classifications of Qi manifested in the body are called the They are Qi, Jing, and Shen. Primal Qi creates the other two forms of Shen and Jing. Qi, Jing and Shen are thought of as air, water, and fire energy respectively. Qi is breath. Jing is associated with water and the kidneys. Shen is the fire and light that lives in our heart and mind.

Torus Field is a donut shape of moving, spiraling, protective energy that surrounds our body, our cells, the earth itself, and our Milky Way galaxy. The torus is the shape of electromagnetic energy.

Triple Warmer has functional meaning as an organ but doesn't have an actual physical location. It controls Qi flow in the body as it ascends and descends, enters and exits, and the entire circulation of body fluid. The Triple Warmer governs the flow of Qi, Shen and Jing. It takes Primal Qi and separates it into its different functions and controls the movement and passage of Qi through Ying Qi or nutritive Qi, Wei Qi or protective Qi, and the blood and bodily fluids. Gathering Qi or Zong Qi is in the upper Warmer. Ying Qi (Nutritive Qi) originates from the Middle Warmer: Wei Qi (Protective Qi) originates from the Lower Warmer.

Uncarved block, Referred to in Lao Tzu's Tao Te Ching. It is free of any markings, the blank canvas, a place of nothingness, of Wuji. This is where creative possibilities arise.

Universal Post a basic stance or posture of Qigong and Tai Chi sometimes called **Hug a Tree**

Vagus nerve is the biggest nerve in the body, sometimes called the wandering nerve. It affects a majority of muscles and the parasympathetic nervous system. About five long exhales can stimulate the vagus nerve and create a state of inner calm and promote healing. When the vagus nerve is stimulated the heart rate slows, blood pressure is lowered, and inflammation and depression is reduced.

Wei Qi is protective Qi which surrounds the body.

Wu were people who lived about 5,000 to 10,000 years ago in the time of matriarchy. It is said the people of the Wu did a ceremonial dance called **Da Wu.**

Wuji a fundamental practice of standing in stillness and alignment. Ideally every Tai Chi form begins with Wuji. The word Wuji is translated as not doing or doing nothing. The classic statement, *"Out of Wuji comes Tai Chi, out of nothing comes something,"* refers to the generative power of Wuji.

Wushu which means Chinese martial arts and are considered a sport. Before the Cultural Revolution they were called Kung Fu or Gong fu which means work accomplished. Gong, work, is like the gong in Qigong, and fu means penetrating heaven. There are three major internal styles of Kung Fu. They are Tai Chi Chuan or Taijiquan, Hsing-i Chuan, and Ba Gua Zhang. Ba Gua is practiced walking in a circle. Hsing-i is practiced in straight lines. Tai Chi is oriented to the Eight Directions as a square within a circle and invokes spiral energy.

> Ba Gua Zhang applies the philosophy of the Eight Directions, the basis of the I Ching. Its name means Eight Trigram Palm. It is considered the deadliest practice in the Chinese martial arts. Although Ba Gua Zhang originated with the "mountain people"

it was designed as a close-quarter combat art. The use of a circular form requires the student to master subtle curvature change while in motion. The student integrates curves and angles into the depth of the sinews and joints and is able to maneuver to easily overtake and neutralize an opponent.

Hsing-i or Xing Yi Quan means Form-Intention Fist or Shape-Will Fist. It refers to the ability of the mind to create an idea and project it into the body. It is considered the most yang of the internal arts.

Wu Xing or the Five Elements regulate nature. Five Element theory is the basis for Traditional Chinese Medicine. In the Yellow Emperor's Classic of Internal Medicine, it is stated that, "The Five Elemental Energies of Wood, Fire, Earth, Metal and Water encompass all the myriad phenomena of nature. It is a paradigm that applies equally to humans" The Five Element combine in various ways in patterns of creation and destruction. The ancient Taoists created a symbol of a pentagram within a circle to represent these patterns.

Wu Shu means "martial art." In 1956 after the Cultural Revolution had begun to settle down, China began to bring Qi Gong, Tai Chi and Gung Fu back into public practice. These martial arts were presented as health or gymnastic exercises and purposely devoid of any spiritual content.

Yongquan An acupuncture point at the bottom of the foot also call the Bubbling Spring which connects our body to the earth energy.

Yi is the power of intention. Yi force gives Qi direction and movement. By our intention, our Yi, we move our Qi to reach our goal. Yi works with our imagination and our creativity. It is the energy we use for the manifestation of our desires. Yi projects the Qi. The basic qigong principle is, "Where the mind goes, the Qi follows." Through our intention, we project and guide the Qi in our own body for healing and can project Qi to heal others. Through Yi we can send and receive Qi.

Yin Yang are the opposing forces of nature, polar-opposites. The Tao produces the pulsating forces of yin (off) and yang (on). Qi energy is always made of yin and yang. Energy is frequency and vibration that move atomic particles and form the elements of our universe. The crest is yang, the trough is yin. Yin-yang are always in harmony. There is no yin without yang.

Ying Qi is nutritive Qi that travels with the blood and keeps the body functioning. It's movement corresponds to the flow of Qi through the organs during each two-hour period of the twenty-four hour day.

Yuan Qi is Primal Energy, the energy of the universe which finds expression in each individual. It is the primordial energy we receive at birth. Yuan Qi is the primal energy of creation, pure harmonious Qi. A quality of Yuan Qi is Loving Light. This can be seen as the universal intelligence or consciousness.

Zazen is a posture of meditation sitting usually on a cushion with your legs crossed and your thumbs lightly touching, left hand supporting the right. This posture gives the best concentration in relative comfort.

RECOMMENDED READING

A Complete Guide to Chi-Gung, Harnessing the Power of the Universe, Daniel Reid, 1998, Simon and Schuster in London.

Heavenly Streams, Meridian Theory in Nei Gong, Damo Mitchell, 2013, Singing Dragon, London.

The Web That Has No Weaver, Understanding Chinese Medicine, Ted J. Kaptchuk O.M.D. 1983, Congdon & Weed.

The Tao of Physics, Fritjof Capra, Shambhala, 1975, Boulder, CO.

Ancient China, Great Ages of Man A History of the World's Cultures by Edward H. Schafer and The Editors of TIME-LIFE BOOKS, 1967

Quantum Healing, Exploring the Frontiers of Mind/Body Medicine Dr. Deepak Chopra, M.D. 1989

The Physics of History by Professor David J. Helfand, Columbia University, Great Courses, 2009.

Lao-Tzu: "My words are very easy to understand" Man-jan Cheng, North Atlantic Books, Berkeley, CA. 1981

Lao Tzu, Tao Te Ching, D.C. Lau, Penguin Books, 1963.

Lao Tzu, Tao Te Ching, A Book about the Way and the Power of the Way, Ursula K. Le Guin, Shambhala, Boston and London, 1998.

The Way of Life, Lao Tzu, Wisdom of Ancient China, R.B. Blakney, A Mentor Book, New York, NY. 1955.

Bodhisattva of Compassion, John Blofield, Shambhala, Boulder, CO. 1978.

Sharp Spear, Crystal Mirror, Martial Arts in Women's Lives, Stephanie T. Hoppe Park Street Press, Rochester, Vermont, 1998.

Taoism, The Parting of the Way, Holmes Welch, Beacon Press, Boston, 1957.

The Study of Qi, in classical texts, Elisabeth Rochat de la Vallee, 2006

A Brief History of Qi, Zhang Yu Huan & Ken Rose, 2001, Paradigm Publications.

The Yellow Emperor's Classic of Medicine, The Essential Text of Chinese Health and Healing, Maoshing NI, Ph.D. 1995, Shambhala Boston and London.

The Tao of Tai-Chi Chuan, Way to Rejuvenation, Jou, Tsung Hwa. 1981, Tai Chi Foundation, Warwick, NY.

The Tarot, A Key to the Wisdom of the Ages, Paul Foster Case, Macy Publishing Company, Richmond, VI. 1947

The Practical Encyclopedia of Feng Shui, Understanding the ancient arts of placement. Gill Hale, 2002 Barnes & Noble Books

101 Miracles of Natural Healing, Luke Chan, Benefactor Press, Rocklin, CA. 2003.

The Complete Idiot's guide to Tai Chi and Qigong Illustrated, Bill Douglas and Angela Wong Douglas, Alpha (Penguin) 2012

Qigong Fever, Body, Science, and Utopia in China, David A. Palmer, Columbia University Press New York, 2007

PYNK QIGONG PRACTICE

1. Feet shoulder width apart, knees bent in same direction as toes, **Wuji,** state of emptiness, not doing, simple standing meditation

2. Alignment with the **Three Powers**: Earth, feel the connection to gravity the root of balance when there is no strain on any part of the body. Feel the gratitude for the food, water and air we receive from earth. Heaven, head touches sky and opens to the expanding creative universe. Feeling we are in the universe and the universe is in us as star dust. Humanity, place hands over lower dan tien, right hand first left hand cover just below navel. Feel your own human form breathing with all of nature.

3. **Whole body breathing**: yin inhale fill, yang exhale empty

4. **Solid and Empty**: weight bearing each foot, bone density strengthening. Bring the minds loving attention into service of the body.

5. Bow in to make a **Qi Field**. Kuan Li, merciful behavior. **Chain Link of Grace** align Dan Tiens.

6. Hands on knees for ROM **Knee Circles** right, ankles and massage feet.

7. Straight legs back flat release hips, **hands on ground** and dangle. Let the weight of the upper body stretch out the legs. Turn to the side open and close waist, center, and turn to other side. Knee circles left. Repeat dangle, organs upside down, blood to brain, relax. Up one vertebra at a time.

8. Feet shoulder width apart **Hip Circles,** massage joints and organs of digestion, elimination, reproduction. Reverse. Feet together,

9. **Waist Circles** cleanse liver and kidneys, both ways.

10. Feet shoulder width, arms hold Qi ball and **Swing,** after a few swings bring one foot out in the direction of eyes, toe in, toe out. Look behind, whole body in spiral energy, twist.

11. **Fly:** throw arms down and pop up back, front, back. Let the weight of the arms and wrists move the body with centrifugal force.

12. Center with arms up, **receive Yuan Qi Primal Qi** from Heaven. Always in perfect harmony.

13. Whole body **scan with Loving Light**, head to feet. Breathe soak in Qi.

14. **Shoulder circles**, thoracic cavity vigor, open and close, harmony, deep breathing massage, reverse.

15. Center in Wuji. Open heart center with feather massage across chest. Place middle finger on lower sternum to **connect to Shen Immortal Spirit** in heart and mind. Feel into evolving consciousness unique and connected to the Universal Consciousness.

16. Eagles beak to tap upper sternum and **stimulate thymus gland and T-cells** to destroy pathogens, viruses, and cancer cells.

17. Massage Kidney point 27 to **harmonize the waters of the body** and toxic release.

18. Massage Lung points 1 and 2 **breathing deeply with all life on this planet** gratefully

19. **Shaman Shake** moving organically subconsciously. Shake out tension. Make noises.

20. Realign to soft center, and extend hands horizontal **extend fingers and contract to fists**

21. Use the mouth of the fist to rub and **nourish kidneys**, adrenal glands and lower back

22. Rub end of tail bone to **stimulate spinal fluid** to nourish your central nervous system

23. From the tailbone up stretch spine pushing the top of the head up and putting space between the vertebrae. Relax hands and arms and make little head circles **Spiraling to Heaven**, both directions. Feel the upper vortex of energy and the Torus Field that surrounds you.

24. Come back to center stand erect and drop your ear towards your shoulder, rotate to chin to shoulder, back to **ear to shoulder** and up to center. Repeat on the other side.

25. Drop your chin towards your chest, feet are grounded, knees are bent, and then look up at the sky, look back and forth and up and down. Drop your **chin to chest**, relax your shoulders, elbows, wrists, and hands. Let any unwanted tension release through the bottom of your feet with the exhale. Face to the sky and make big circles with your eyes. Return to center.

26. Drop your chin towards your chest and make **large head rolls**, leaning back so you don't hurt your vertebrae. Let any tension drift away.

27. Come back to center and open palms, feel the **whole body relaxed but alert**, feel the inner smile deep inside and your natural state of contentment. Three deep breaths. All is Well!

28. Fists in front of shoulders, elbow in to open the back. Articulate fingers, **little finger out** followed by each finger stretching out, little finger in return to fist.

29. Place the heels of your hands over your ears to block out sounds and flick your middle finger off your index finger to create a clicking thumping sound and concentrate on harmonizing the endocrine system sending vibration into the Pituitary gland, **Celestial Drumming**. After about 30 seconds pop the hands off the ears and feel the harmony.

30. Feet shoulder width apart, your palms face down to the earth. **Sinking Qi** into the earth, exhale completely. Inhale as you expand Qi, allow your wrists to rise up to about shoulder level. Hold your breath as your palms face each other and condense Qi as you Gather the Qi ball between your hands with your arms stretched out at heart level. Receive Qi as you bring the Qi ball towards the solar plexus and exhale as you sink the Qi down again, receiving Qi through the lower dan tien and then sink into the earth. Repeat three times.

31. Return to center. Shift the weight to the right foot and bring the left toe in with the exhale. Inhale and lift the left knee up, Crane Stands on One Leg, exhale down. Inhale lift the arms over the head, back of the hands together as the **Crane Spreads**

its Wings. Reach out to the sides, sink down and shift the weight to the left foot and repeat each side for balance practice. Repeat several times. Come to center, bringing the hands to the lower dan tien and take a few breathes harmonize the Qi.

32. Bow out to **close Qi Field** in gratitude, Kuan Li, Merciful Behavior, for yourself, for others, and for all of nature. Thank all teachers that have given us these healing forms.

Give yourself some Qi love every day!

Simu Janet Seaforth
Po Yun Nei Kuan
Cloverdale, CA. 95425
2021